THE STORAGE OF
FLAMMABLE
LIQUIDS
IN TANKS

HSE BOOKS

First published 1998

Note: material previously contained in *The storage of flammable liquids in fixed tanks (up to 10 000m^3 total capacity)* HSG50 1990 and *The storage of flammable liquids in fixed tanks (exceeding 10 000m^3 total capacity)* HSG52 1991

ISBN 0 7176 1470 0

CONTENTS

INTRODUCTION

General

1   This book gives guidance on the design, construction, operation and maintenance of installations used for the storage of flammable liquids in fixed tanks operating at or near atmospheric pressure. It applies to new installations and to existing installations where reasonably practicable. It replaces HSG50 *The storage of flammable liquids in fixed tanks (up to 10 000 m³ total capacity)* and HSG52 *The storage of flammable liquids in fixed tanks (exceeding 10 000 m³ total capacity).*

2   The guidance is aimed at managers and supervisors involved in storing flammable liquids. It is relevant to many industries such as:

- chemical;

- petrochemical;

- paints;

- solvents;

- pharmaceutical.

It may also be of interest to designers and installers. Trade organisations may wish to use the guidance as a basis for more specific guidance for their own members.

3   This book gives help in the assessment of the risks arising from the storage of flammable liquids, and it describes measures to control those risks. Assessment, by employers and the self-employed, of the risks to workers and others who may be affected by their activities is one of the requirements of the Management of Health and Safety at Work Regulations 1992[1,2,3]. This publication also advises on how to comply with the relevant parts of the Health and Safety at Work etc Act 1974[4,5,6] and the Highly Flammable Liquids and Liquefied Petroleum Gases Regulations 1972[7-13], and with other relevant legislation.

4   Legal requirements, guidance and the standards referred to in this guidance are listed in the reference section. They are subject to amendment from time to time. Where a British Standard is quoted, any other national or international standard which provides an equivalent level of safety is acceptable. The glossary at the back of this book explains the particular terms used in this guidance.

Scope of this document

What this guidance applies to

5   This guidance applies to flammable liquids with a flashpoint of 55°C or below. This includes all highly flammable liquids (as defined by the Highly Flammable Liquids and Liquefied Petroleum Gases Regulations 1972[7]) and all petroleum spirit and petroleum mixtures as defined in the Petroleum (Consolidation Act) 1928[14] and the Petroleum (Mixtures) Order 1929[15]. It includes all liquids that are classified as flammable, highly flammable or extremely flammable for supply according to CHIP: Chemicals (Hazard Information and Packaging for Supply) Regulations 1996[16-20].

6   The guidance is also relevant to liquids with a flashpoint above 55°C which are stored at temperatures above their flashpoint.

7   Some of the precautions described may not be necessary for liquids with a flashpoint in the range 32°-55°C and stored at ambient temperature. Advice on less restrictive measures for these liquids is given in paragraphs 223-235. Where no variation is given, the advice in the main text applies.

8   The guidance applies to above and below ground fixed bulk storage tanks. It applies to premises where flammable liquids are stored in individual tanks or groups of tanks. It may also be applied to portable or skid mounted vessels with capacities in excess of 1000 litres.

9   Advice is provided on transfer facilities for road and rail loading and unloading.

What the guidance does not apply to

10   The guidance does not apply to:

- flammable liquids stored in portable containers and drums with capacities of 1000 litres or less. These are covered by HSG51 *The storage of flammable liquids in containers*[8]. Generally, the storage of flammable liquids in fixed bulk tanks is preferable to storage of the same quantity in drums or similar containers, as spillage during handling is reduced;

- liquids with a flashpoint between 21°C and 55°C but which do not support combustion when tested at 55°C, in the manner described in Schedule 2 of the Highly Flammable Liquids and Liquefied Petroleum Gases Regulations 1972[7];

- flammable liquids which present special hazards requiring specific storage conditions, such as ethylene oxide, peroxides, and other liquids which entail a risk of rapid decomposition, polymerisation or spontaneous combustion;

- petroleum kept in fixed tanks at retail filling stations. Guidance on filling stations and similar private premises is available in HSG146 *Dispensing petrol: Assessing and controlling the risk of fire and explosion at sites where petrol is stored and dispensed as a fuel*[21];

- carriage of flammable liquids (on or off site), including temporary storage at lorry parks and transit areas;

- liquefied petroleum gas and other substances which are gases at ambient temperature and pressure but are stored as liquids under pressure or refrigeration;

- flammable liquids stored under pressure. In these cases the guidance on LPG storage[22] may be appropriate;

- vessels, which are an integral part of process plant;

- loading and unloading of ships. This is covered by Guidance Note GS40 *The loading and unloading of flammable liquids and gases at harbours and inland waterways*[23,24].

11   Released vapours arising from the storage of flammable liquids can have environmental consequences and may be subject to controls under the Environmental Protection Act 1990[25,26,27]. Although this guidance does not attempt to cover environmental issues, the advice it contains for the safe storage of flammable liquids will also provide protection for the environment. Further guidance is available from the Environment Agency, the Scottish Environmental Protection Agency or from local authorities, who enforce the Environmental Protection Act.

12   Flammable liquids can also pose a health hazard if they are inhaled, ingested or come into contact with skin or eyes. Information on the health hazards of a particular liquid, and on any specific precautions required, should be obtained from the safety data sheet[17] or from the supplier. The Control of Substances Hazardous to Health Regulations 1988[28,29] require employers to assess the risks from exposure to hazardous substances and the precautions needed.

The storage of flammable liquids in tanks

FIRE AND EXPLOSION HAZARDS

13   The main hazards associated with the storage and handling of flammable liquids are fire and explosion, involving either the liquid or the vapour given off from it. Fires and explosions are likely to occur when vapour or liquid is released accidentally or deliberately into areas where there may be an ignition source, or when an ignition source is introduced into an area where there may be flammable atmospheres.

14   Common causes of such incidents include:

- inadequate design and installation of equipment;

- inadequate inspection and maintenance;

- failure or malfunction of equipment;

- lack of awareness of the properties of flammable liquids;

- operator error, due to lack of training;

- exposure to heat from a nearby fire;

- inadequate control of ignition sources;

- electrostatic discharges;

- heating materials above their auto-ignition temperature;

- dismantling or disposing of equipment containing flammable liquids;

- hot work on or close to flammable liquid vessels.

15   Combustion of liquids occurs when flammable vapours released from the surface of the liquid ignite. The amount of flammable vapour given off from a liquid, and therefore the extent of the fire or explosion hazard, depends largely on the temperature of the liquid, how much of the surface area is exposed, how long it is exposed for, and the air movement over the surface. The hazard also depends on the physical properties of the liquid such as flashpoint, auto-ignition temperature, viscosity, and the upper and lower explosion limits.

16   The flashpoint is the lowest temperature at which a flammable liquid gives off vapour in sufficient quantity to form a combustible mixture with air near the surface of the liquid. Generally, a liquid with a flashpoint below the ambient temperature will give off sufficient flammable vapour which when mixed with air can be ignited. Liquids with a flashpoint greater than ambient temperature are less likely to give off flammable concentrations of vapours unless they are heated, mixed with low flashpoint materials or released under pressure as a mist or a spray. However, a material above its flashpoint can be easily ignited if it is spread out as a thin film over a large area or spilled on to clothing or insulation.

17   The viscosity of the liquid is also significant as it determines how far any spilt material will spread and therefore the size of any exposed surface. Solvents generally have a low viscosity and when spilt spread quickly, allowing a rapid build-up of vapours from the surface of the liquid. Also vapours can drift or be blown away from the surface of the liquid - if the vapours are ignited the flame will travel or 'flash back' to the liquid.

18   As mentioned in paragraph 12, flammable liquids can also pose health and environmental hazards. Further information should be obtained from the safety data sheet or from the supplier.

LEGAL
REQUIREMENTS

19   The Highly Flammable Liquids and Liquefied Petroleum Gases Regulations 1972[7] require precautions to reduce the risk of fires and explosions, where flammable liquids or gases are stored or processed. These precautions include measures to prevent leaks, spills and dangerous concentrations of vapours, and to control ignition sources.

20   Under the Management of Health and Safety at Work Regulations 1992[1,2], every employer has a duty to carry out an assessment of the risks to the health and safety of employees and of anyone who may be affected by the work activity. This is so that the necessary preventive and protective measures can be identified and implemented.

21   If the installation is subject to the Control of Industrial Major Accident Hazard (CIMAH) Regulations 1984[31,32,33], then the person in control of the industrial activity is required to demonstrate that the major accident hazards have been identified and that the activity is being operated safely. For larger inventories, the requirements will include the submission of a written safety report, preparation of an on-site emergency plan and provision of certain information for the public. These regulations are expected to be replaced in February 1999 by the Control of Major Accident Hazards Involving Dangerous Substances (COMAH) Regulations.

22   There are also general duties under health and safety law which are relevant. Further information on legal requirements is given in Appendix 1.

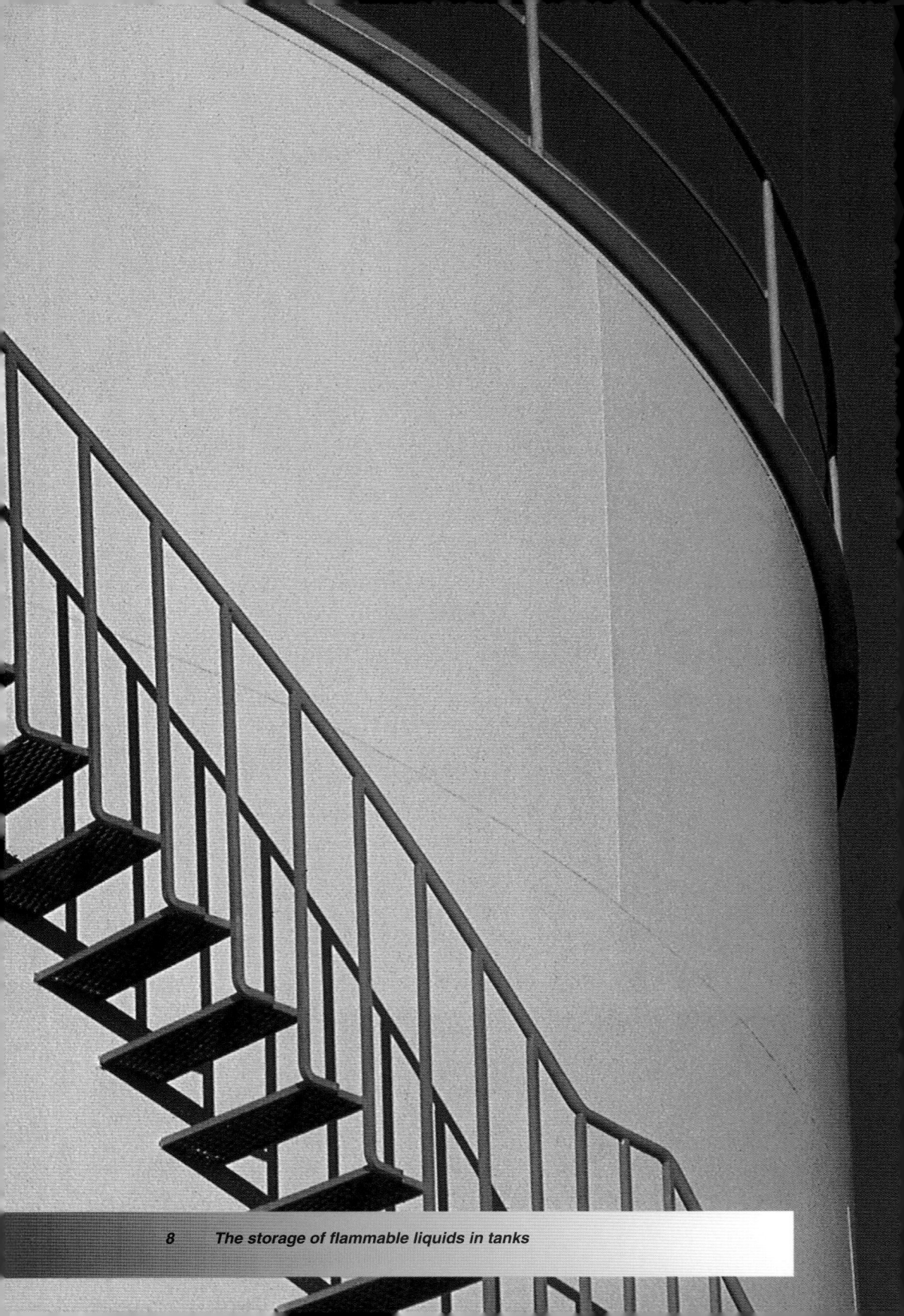

The storage of flammable liquids in tanks

RISK ASSESSMENT

23   HSE recommends a five step approach to risk assessment[3]:

Step 1:   **look for the hazards;**

Step 2:   **decide who might be harmed, and how seriously;**

Step 3:   **evaluate the risks arising from the hazards and decide whether existing precautions are adequate or more should be done;**

Step 4:   **record your findings (this is a statutory requirement if you have five or more employees);**

Step 5:   **review your assessment from time to time and revise it if necessary.**

24   The assessment should include risks arising from the tank, and risks to the tank from external sources. The aims of the assessment are to:

- minimise the risk of a spillage of flammable liquid;

- minimise the risk of a fire or explosion occurring at the tank itself;

- mitigate the consequences of such an incident, particularly with regard to people and the environment;

- protect the tank from fires occurring elsewhere.

25   Factors which should be considered when assessing a storage installation include:

- storage capacity;

- location of the tank, in relation to site boundaries, buildings, process areas and fixed sources of ignition;

- design standards for the installation;

- quantities and locations of other flammable liquids;

- quantities and locations of other dangerous substances;

- activities on adjacent premises;

- training and supervision of site operatives;

- frequency of deliveries;

- loading and unloading operations;

- inspection and maintenance.

26   Risk assessments should be carried out prior to the installation of new facilities, modification of existing facilities and the demolition of obsolete facilities. It is advisable to seek the advice of organisations such as the fire authority, the Environment Agency, the Health and Safety Executive and insurance companies.

27   The overriding concern, in the event of a fire or explosion involving a storage tank, is to ensure that people are able to escape to safety.

Control measures

28   You will need to know what is good practice to help you decide if your precautions and control measures are sufficient, and that the risk is as low as is reasonably practicable. This section will briefly describe control measures for the storage of flammable liquids. More detailed information is supplied in later sections of the book.

Containment

29   Flammable liquids should be stored in tanks or containers constructed to a national or international standard to ensure their strength and integrity. Further information is given in paragraphs 61-68.

30   There should also be means to contain spillage and prevent it spreading to other parts of the premises. Information on bunding is given in paragraphs 137-152.

Separation

31   Separation is an important means of providing protection for tanks containing flammable liquids. Separation has particular advantages because not only does it protect people and property from the effects of a fire at the tank, but it also protects the tank from fires which may occur elsewhere on site. Further advice on the recommended separation distances is given in paragraphs 46-55.

Ventilation

32   Good ventilation ensures that any flammable vapours given off from a spill, leak or release will be rapidly dispersed. This may be achieved by locating storage tanks, transfer facilities, vent pipes etc in the open air, in a well-ventilated position.

Substitution

33   In some instances, such as at production sites, it may be possible to eliminate or reduce the quantity of flammable liquid on site. For some processes, higher-flashpoint or water-based products are now available. It may be practicable to reduce the storage inventory by better planning and stock control, by maintaining smaller buffer stocks and by removing from site any materials which are no longer used in the process.

Control of ignition sources

34   In certain areas, flammable atmospheres may occur either during normal operation or due to accidental spills or leakage. These areas are called hazardous areas, and measures to control the introduction of sources of ignition are required in these areas. Common ignition sources include:

- unprotected electrical equipment;

- naked flames including welding and cutting equipment;

- smoking materials;

- vehicles with internal combustion engines;

- hot surfaces;

- frictional heating or sparking;

- static electricity.

35   Hazardous area classification is the method used to identify areas where flammable concentrations of gases or vapours are likely to be present. The aim is to reduce to a minimum acceptable level the probability of a flammable atmosphere coinciding with an electrical or other ignition source. It is normally used to select fixed electrical equipment, but it can also be used in the control of other potential ignition sources such as portable electrical equipment, hot surfaces and vehicles. Advice is available in:

- British Standard BS EN 60079-10: 1996 *Electrical apparatus for explosive atmospheres, Part 10: Classification of hazardous areas*[34]; and

- Institute of Petroleum (IP) *Area classification code for petroleum installations: model code of safe practice in the petroleum industry part 15*[35].

36   There are three classes of hazardous area or zone: zone 0, zone 1 and zone 2. A zone is an area around a process or activity where a flammable atmosphere may be present. The definitions of the three hazardous zones, according to British Standard, BS EN 60079-10 are given in Table 1.

Table 1 Definition of zones

Zone	Definition
Zone 0	An area in which an explosive gas mixture is continuously present or present for long periods.
Zone 1	An area in which an explosive gas mixture is likely to occur in normal operation.
Zone 2	An area in which an explosive gas mixture is not likely to occur in normal operation, and, if it does occur, is likely to do so only infrequently and will exist for a short period only.

37   The extent of the zones will depend on:

- ventilation;

- design of the tank;

- the source of the release;

- the flashpoint; and

- vapour density.

Figure 1 Vertical storage tank - typical hazardous area classification

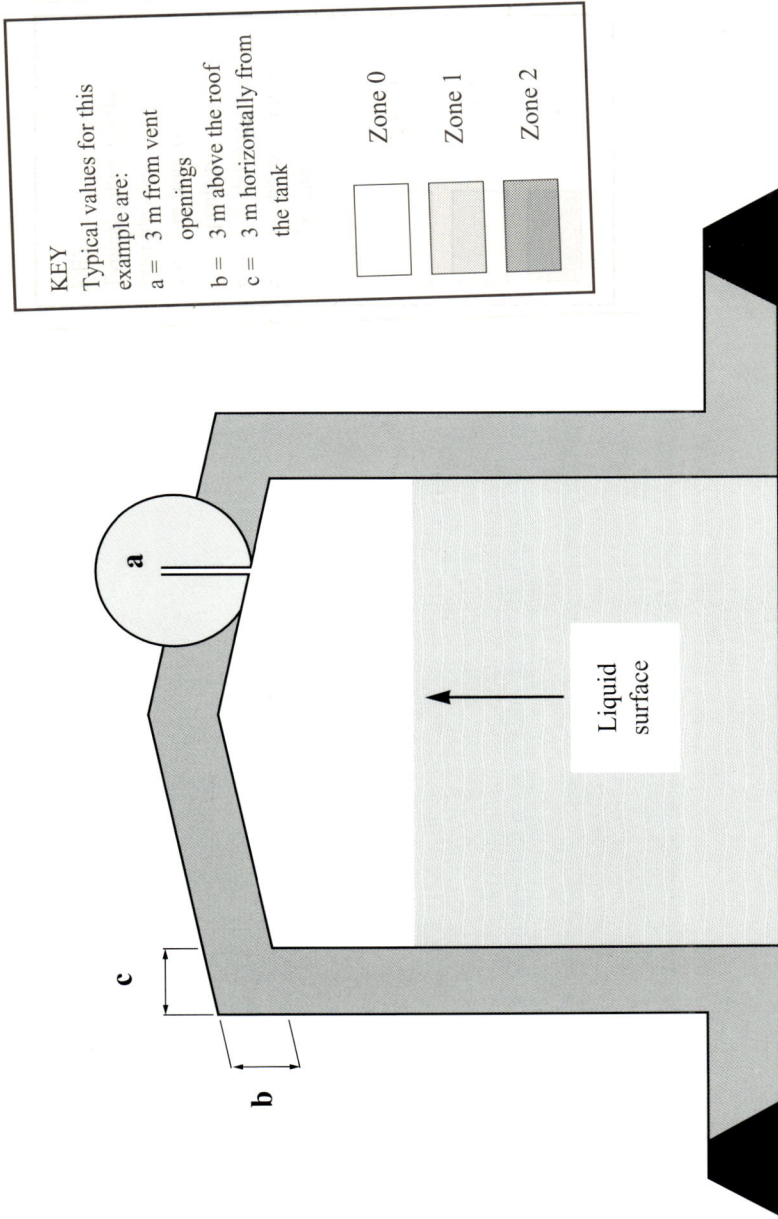

KEY
Typical values for this
example are:
a = 3 m from vent
      openings
b = 3 m above the roof
c = 3 m horizontally from
      the tank

Zone 0

Zone 1

Zone 2

Liquid
surface

a

c

b

Examples of hazardous area classification for a fixed-roof tank and a tanker filling installation are shown in Figures 1 and 2. These examples are for general guidance only, as local conditions should always be taken into account when carrying out a classification.

38   Where reasonably practicable, electrical equipment should be installed in non-hazardous areas. Where this cannot be done, equipment should be selected, installed and maintained in accordance with BS 5345 *Code of practice for the selection, installation and maintenance of electrical apparatus for use in potentially explosive atmospheres*[36] (or other equivalent standard).

39   When a hazardous area classification has been carried out, the location of the zones should be recorded on a plan. This may then be used to prevent sources of ignition being brought into hazardous areas.

Figure 2 Tanker filling installation for highly flammable liquids - typical hazardous area classification

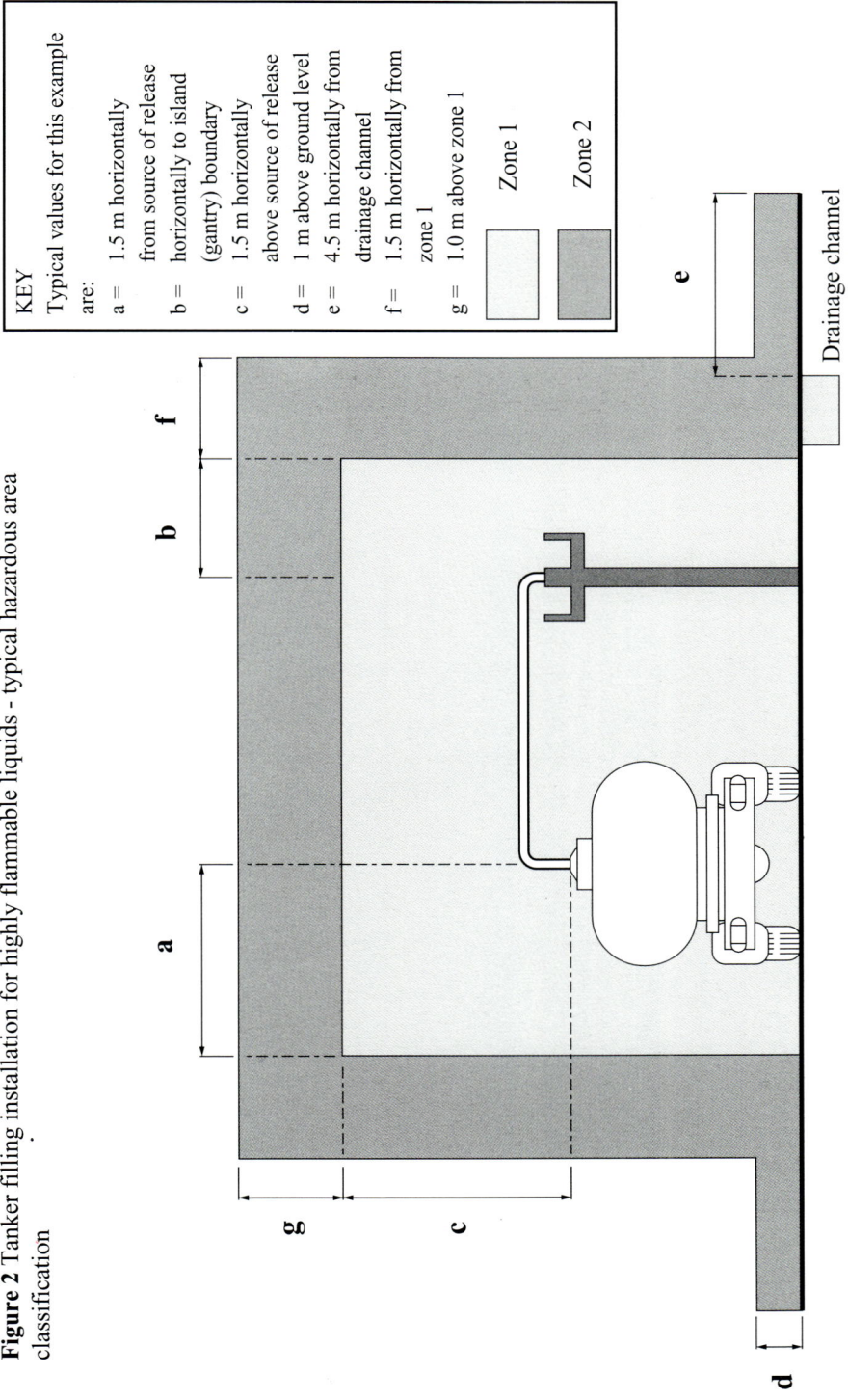

KEY

Typical values for this example are:

a = 1.5 m horizontally from source of release

b = horizontally to island (gantry) boundary

c = 1.5 m horizontally above source of release

d = 1 m above ground level

e = 4.5 m horizontally from drainage channel

f = 1.5 m horizontally from zone 1

g = 1.0 m above zone 1

Zone 1

Zone 2

Drainage channel

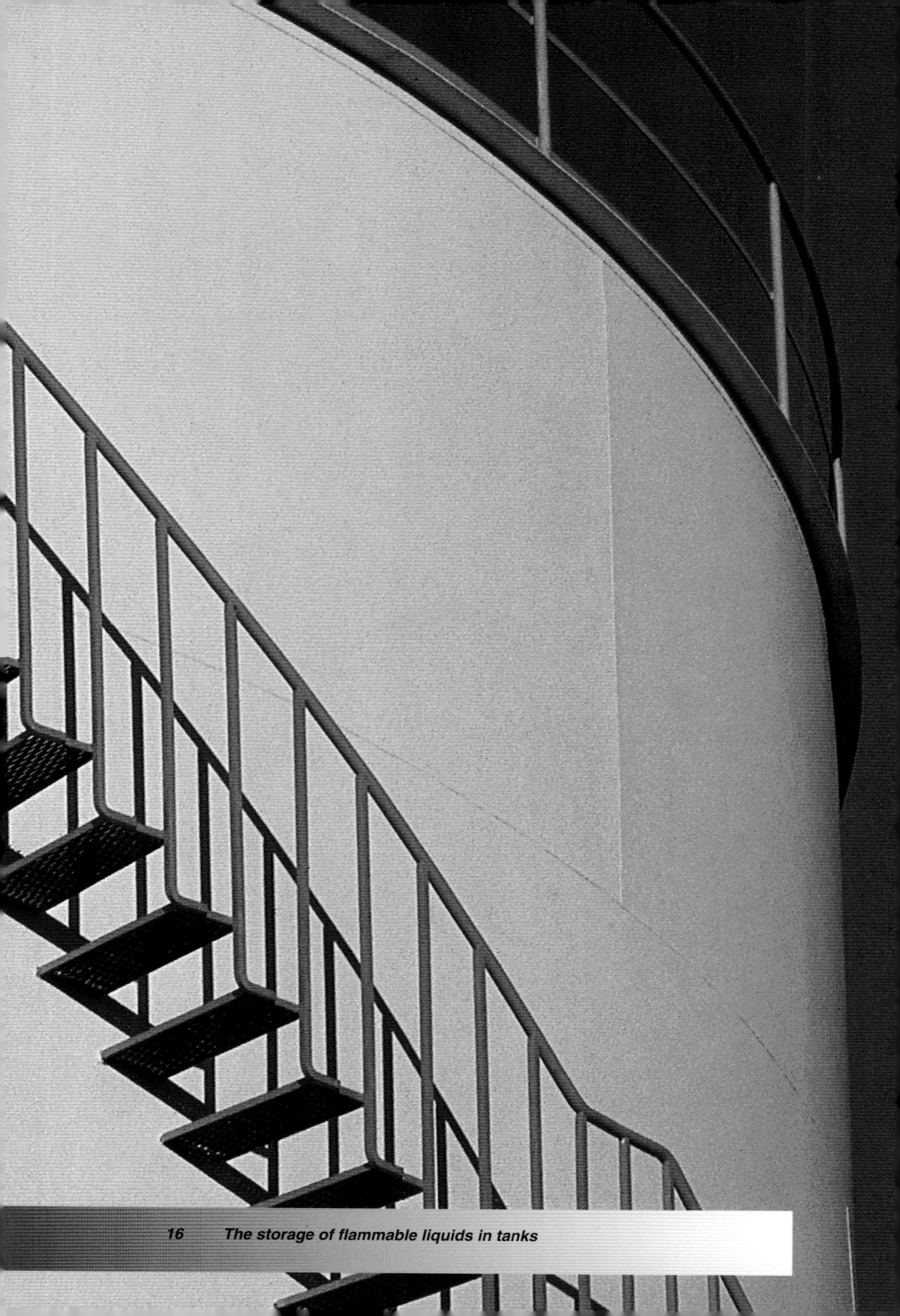

The storage of flammable liquids in tanks

LOCATION AND LAYOUT OF TANKS

General

40   The location and layout of a storage installation should be selected with care. The aims are to protect people and property from the effects of a fire at the tank, and to protect the tank from fires which may occur elsewhere on site. As a rule, if the temperature of a steel tank is allowed to rise above 300°C, then the structure of the tank will be adversely affected and it may rupture.

41   Storage tanks may be located above ground, underground or in mounds. Each location has different advantages and disadvantages. Storage at ground level, in the open air, has advantages because leaks are more readily detected and contained, and any vapour produced will normally be dissipated by natural ventilation. Examinations, modifications and repairs are also easier, and corrosion can be more readily identified and controlled.

42   Underground or mounded tanks give better fire protection and save space. But leakage, resulting from damage or corrosion, may be difficult to detect. This could lead to ground contamination, environmental problems and possible fire and explosion risks to nearby buildings and basements.

43   When selecting the location of a single or multi-tank installation, consideration should be given to the distance of the proposed storage from:

- the site boundary;

- on-site buildings, particularly those that are occupied;

- fixed ignition sources;

- storage or processing of other dangerous substances;

- road or rail tanker transfer facilities.

44   Other factors to consider are:

- the position of the tanks (above ground or below ground);

- the size and capacity of the tanks;

- the design of the tanks (fixed roof or floating roof).

45   Tanks should not be located:

- under buildings;

- on the roofs of buildings;

- in positions raised high above ground level;

- on top of one another;

- above tunnels, culverts or sewers.

Tank locations inside buildings should be avoided (but see paragraphs 56-59).

Tanks above ground

46   Tanks above ground should be sited in a well-ventilated position separated from the site boundary, occupied buildings, sources of ignition, and process areas. Figure 3 shows a plan of a typical layout for storage tanks. The layout of tanks should always take into account the accessibility needed for the emergency services.

47   The separation distances will depend on various factors but primarily on the capacity of the tank. Advice on separation distances is given for 'small' tanks, generally associated with small to medium chemical processes, and for 'large' tanks associated with refinery and other large-scale storage facilities.

48   The separation distances given are unlikely to give complete protection in the event of a fire or explosion involving the tank, but should allow sufficient time for people to be evacuated, provided there are good means of escape. They should also allow sufficient time for additional fire-fighting equipment and emergency procedures to be mobilised.

49   Under certain circumstances, it may be necessary to increase the separation distances or provide additional fire protection. Such circumstances may include:

- where there are problems with the local water supply;

Figure 3 General layout of storage tanks showing separation distances

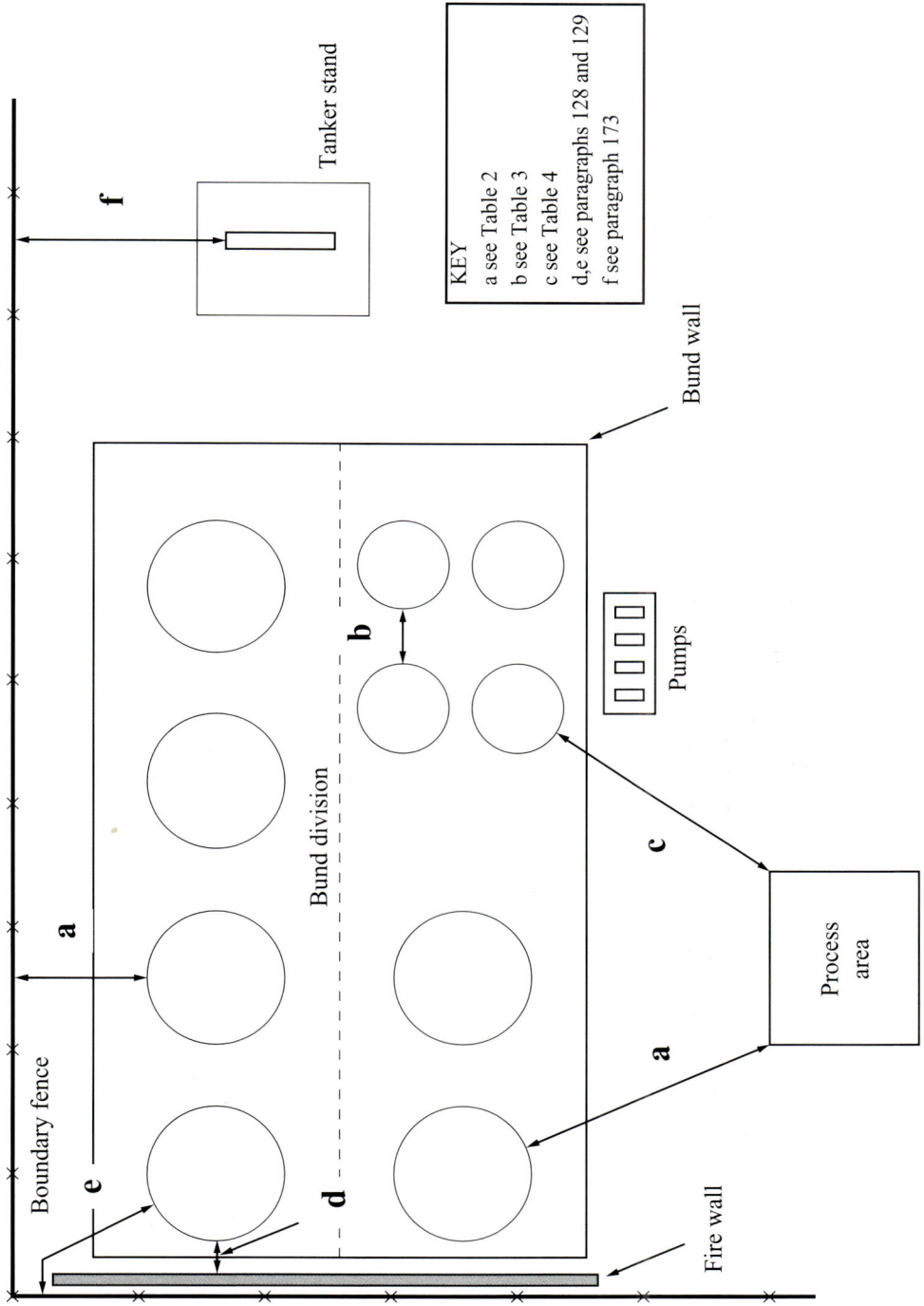

KEY
a see Table 2
b see Table 3
c see Table 4
d,e see paragraphs 128 and 129
f see paragraph 173

Tanker stand

Bund wall

Pumps

Bund division

Process area

Boundary fence

Fire wall

- where the site is remote from external help (such as the fire authority);

- where the tank is close to a heavily populated area.

Separation distances for 'small' tanks

50   For the purposes of this guidance 'small' tanks are considered to be tanks with a diameter of less than 10 m. Table 2 shows the minimum recommended separation distances for single 'small' tanks. The distances are based on what is considered to be good practice and have been widely accepted by industry. The minimum separation distance is the minimum distance between any point on the tank and any building, boundary, process unit, or fixed source of ignition.

Table 2 Minimum recommended separation distances for single 'small' tanks, from site boundaries, buildings, process areas and fixed sources of ignition

Tank capacity (m³)	Separation distance (m)
Less than or equal to 1	1*
Greater than 1 and less than or equal to 5	4
Greater than 5 and less than or equal to 33	6
Greater than 33 and less than or equal to 100	8
Greater than 100 and less than or equal to 250	10
Greater than 250	15

* But at least 2 m from doors, plain-glazed windows, or other openings or means of escape. Also not below any opening (including building eaves and means of escape) from an upper floor, regardless of vertical distance.

Separation distances for groups of 'small' tanks

51   Small tanks may be placed together in groups. A tank is considered as part of a group if adjacent tanks are within the separation distances given in Table 2. The aggregate capacity of the group should be no more than 8000 m³ and the tanks should be arranged so that they are all accessible for fire-fighting purposes.

52   The recommended minimum separation distances between individual tanks in a group are given in Table 3. If a serious fire develops involving one tank in a group then it is unlikely that these between-tank separation distances will prevent damage or even destruction of the adjacent tanks. However, they should allow sufficient time for emergency procedures to be implemented and for people to be evacuated from areas threatened by the incident.

Table 3 Minimum between-tank separation distances for groups of 'small' tanks

Tank size	Recommended separation distance between tanks
Less than or equal to 100 m^3	The minimum required for safe construction and operation
Greater than 100 m^3 but less than 10 m in diameter	Equal to or greater than 2 m

53   For the purpose of determining separation distances from site boundaries, buildings, process areas and fixed sources of ignition, a group of small tanks may be regarded as one tank. The minimum recommended separation distances for groups of small tanks are given in Table 4. The minimum recommended separation distance between adjacent groups of small tanks is 15 m.

Table 4 Minimum recommended separation distances for groups of 'small' tanks from site boundaries, buildings, process areas and fixed sources of ignition

Total capacity of the group (m^3)	Separation distance (m)
Less than or equal to 3	1*
Greater than 3 and less than or equal to 15	4
Greater than 15 and less than or equal to 100	6
Greater than 100 and less than or equal to 300	8
Greater than 300 and less than or equal to 750	10
Greater than 750 and less than or equal to 8000	15

*But at least 2 m from doors, plain-glazed windows, or other openings or means of escape. Also not below any opening (including building eaves and means of escape) from an upper floor, regardless of vertical distance.

Separation distances for 'large' tanks

54   The minimum recommended separation distances for 'large' tanks are given in Table 5. The table is based on the IP *Fire precautions at petroleum refineries and bulk storage installations: model code of safe practice part 19*[37].

Table 5 Minimum separation distances for 'large' tanks

Factor	Minimum separation from any part of the tank

Between adjacent fixed-roof tanks	Equal to the smaller of the following:
	   (a) the diameter of the smaller tank;
	   (b) half the diameter of the larger tank;
	   (c) 15 m;
	but not less than 10 m

Between adjacent floating-roof tanks	10 m for tanks up to and including 45 m diameter 15 m for tanks over 45 m diameter The spacing is determined by the size of the larger tank

Between a floating-roof tank and a fixed-roof tank	Equal to the smaller of the following:
	   (a) the diameter of the smaller tank;
	   (b) half the diameter of the larger tank;
	   (c) 15 m;
	but not less than 10 m

Between a group of small tanks and any tank outside the group	15 m
Between a tank and the site boundary, any designated non-hazardous area, process area or any fixed source of ignition	15 m

Separation from other dangerous substances

55 Separation may also be used to prevent or delay the spread of fire to and from storage or process areas where other dangerous substances may be present in quantity. Table 6 shows the minimum recommended separation distances from LPG storage[22,38]. Table 2 may be used to estimate separation distances from other hazardous substances. If published guidance exists, for the particular hazardous substance concerned, the recommended minimum separation distance is the greater of the distances given in Table 2 and the relevant guidance.

Table 6 Minimum recommended separation distance from LPG storage

	LPG cylinders (>50 kg total capacity)	LPG vessels (up to 135 m³)	LPG vessel (over 135 m³)
Flammable liquid (flashpoint <32°C)	3 m to bund wall	6 m to bund wall	15 m to bund wall
Flammable liquid (flashpoint 32°C - 65°C) Tank size up to 3 m³	3 m to bund wall	3 m to bund wall	6 m to bund wall
Flammable liquid (flashpoint 32°C - 65°C) Tank size over 3 m³	3 m to bund wall	3 m to bund wall	15 m to bund wall

Storage of flammable liquids in buildings

56   Flammable liquids should not normally be stored in bulk tanks in buildings. If storage is required in buildings then only the minimum amount should be stored and for the minimum time, preferably no more than that needed for one day or one shift.

57   Additional safety measures may be needed for the building. These include:

- a single-storey and generally non-combustible construction;

- a lightweight roof or other means of explosion relief. Where this is not reasonably practicable an acceptable alternative is to provide sufficient mechanical ventilation to remove flammable vapour released in the event of an incident;

- a high standard of natural ventilation, using high and low-level openings in the walls (typically 2.5% of the total wall and roof area) leading directly to the open air. Alternatively, permanent mechanical ventilation can be used, equivalent to at least five air changes per hour[39];

- fire separation (by means of a partition of at least 30 minutes fire resistance) between the part of the building housing the tank and other parts of the building, or other buildings within 4 m; and

- adequate means of escape.

58   The tank should have the following features:

- effective means of preventing the spread of leakage. Where appropriate the building walls may form part of the bund, providing they are impervious, have sufficient strength and doorways are fitted with kerbs, ramps or sills;

- vents which discharge to a safe place in the open air.

59   Adequate means of cooling the tank surface in the event of fire in the building may be needed. In some cases this may be done by the fire brigade using portable equipment, but in others a fixed water installation may be necessary. Adequate drainage is essential to avoid tank flotation and local flooding.

Underground tanks

60   The minimum recommended separation distance from any underground tank to any building line is at least 2 m, to avoid undermining the building foundations. It is advisable to increase this distance to 6 m for a basement or pit, to minimise the risk of vapour accumulation.

DESIGN AND CONSTRUCTION

The design of the tank

61   To ensure mechanical integrity, storage tanks should be designed and constructed in accordance with a British or European standard or any other national or international standard that provides an equivalent level of safety. Standards[40-44] which may be applicable include:

- BS 2594 *Carbon steel welded horizontal cylindrical storage tanks;*

- BS 2654 *Manufacture of vertical steel welded non-refrigerated storage tanks with butt-welded shells for the petroleum industry;*

- BS 4994 *Design and construction of vessels and tanks in reinforced plastics.*

62   Draft European standards[45,46] are in preparation:

- prEN 265001 *Specification for the design and manufacture of site-built, vertical, cylindrical, flat-bottomed, above-ground, welded, metallic tanks for the storage of liquids at ambient temperature;*

- prEN 976 *Underground tanks of GRP - Horizontal cylindrical tanks for the non-pressure storage of liquid petroleum based fuels.*

63   The materials used in the construction of the tank or, where appropriate, the tank lining, should be compatible with the chemical and physical properties of the liquid, to ensure that no interaction occurs which might cause failure of the tank.

64   Above-ground tanks are generally constructed of steel or other material which can withstand for a short period the effects of direct flame impingement or radiant heat from a fire in the vicinity. If GRP (glass reinforced plastic) tanks are installed above ground, then they may need additional precautions to ensure that their integrity is not lost rapidly in the event of fire.

65   Where a manhole is fitted to a tank the manhole should be at least 460 mm inside diameter. For tanks over 2 m in diameter and for tanks where personnel may have to wear protective clothing and breathing apparatus for entry, the manhole should be at least 600 mm inside diameter.

66   If the tank is to be heated, additional precautions may be needed. These are outlined in paragraphs 162-170.

67   Tanks may be compartmented. Different materials should not be stored in the same tank, if leakage from one compartment to another is likely to cause a hazard. Mixing of chemically incompatible materials may cause an unwanted and possibly dangerous reaction within the tank. Even accidental mixing of apparently compatible solvents may create a hazard if the contaminated solvent is then fed into a process.

68   Figures 4 and 5 show examples of horizontal and vertical tank installations. Figure 6 shows a typical underground tank installation.

Double skin storage tanks

69   A double skin storage tank could be considered as a tank within a tank. The space between the tanks is kept to a minimum and is used to provide a means of monitoring the soundness of both the inner and outer skin. The monitoring system is an intrinsically safe system using either liquid level, vacuum, or pressure to provide an alarm if one of the skins fails. This is of particular benefit for tanks below ground.

Corrosion protection

70   Corrosion is one of the main causes of equipment failure. It can occur both internally and externally at any exposed metal surface. Protection may be provided by paints or other coatings. BS 5493 *Code of practice for protective coating of iron and steel structures against corrosion*[47] gives guidance on the various methods that may be used. Cathodic protection may be used as an additional precaution[48].

71   Chemical-resistant coatings or paints are available. These are generally sprayed on in several layers to the required thickness. Coatings should be inspected for thickness, continuity and hardness prior to installing the tank. For underground tanks, a bituminous coating can be applied using the following standards:

- BS 3416 *Bitumen-based coating solutions for cold application, suitable for use in contact with potable water*[49]; or

- BS 6949 *Bitumen-based coatings for cold application, excluding use in contact with potable water*[50].

Figure 4 Typical horizontal storage tank (top discharge)

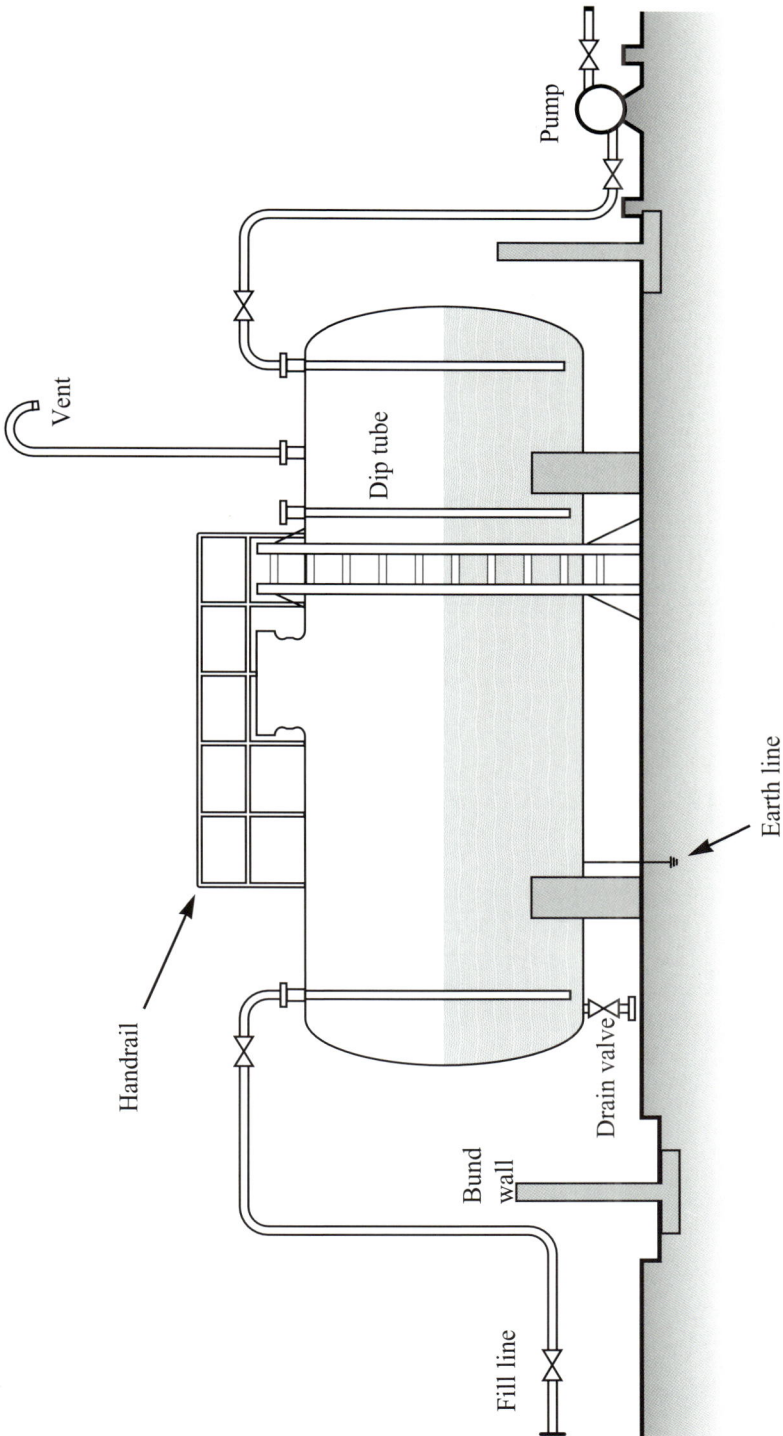

Pump

Vent

Dip tube

Earth line

Handrail

Bund wall

Drain valve

Fill line

Figure 5 Typical vertical storage tank (top filled)

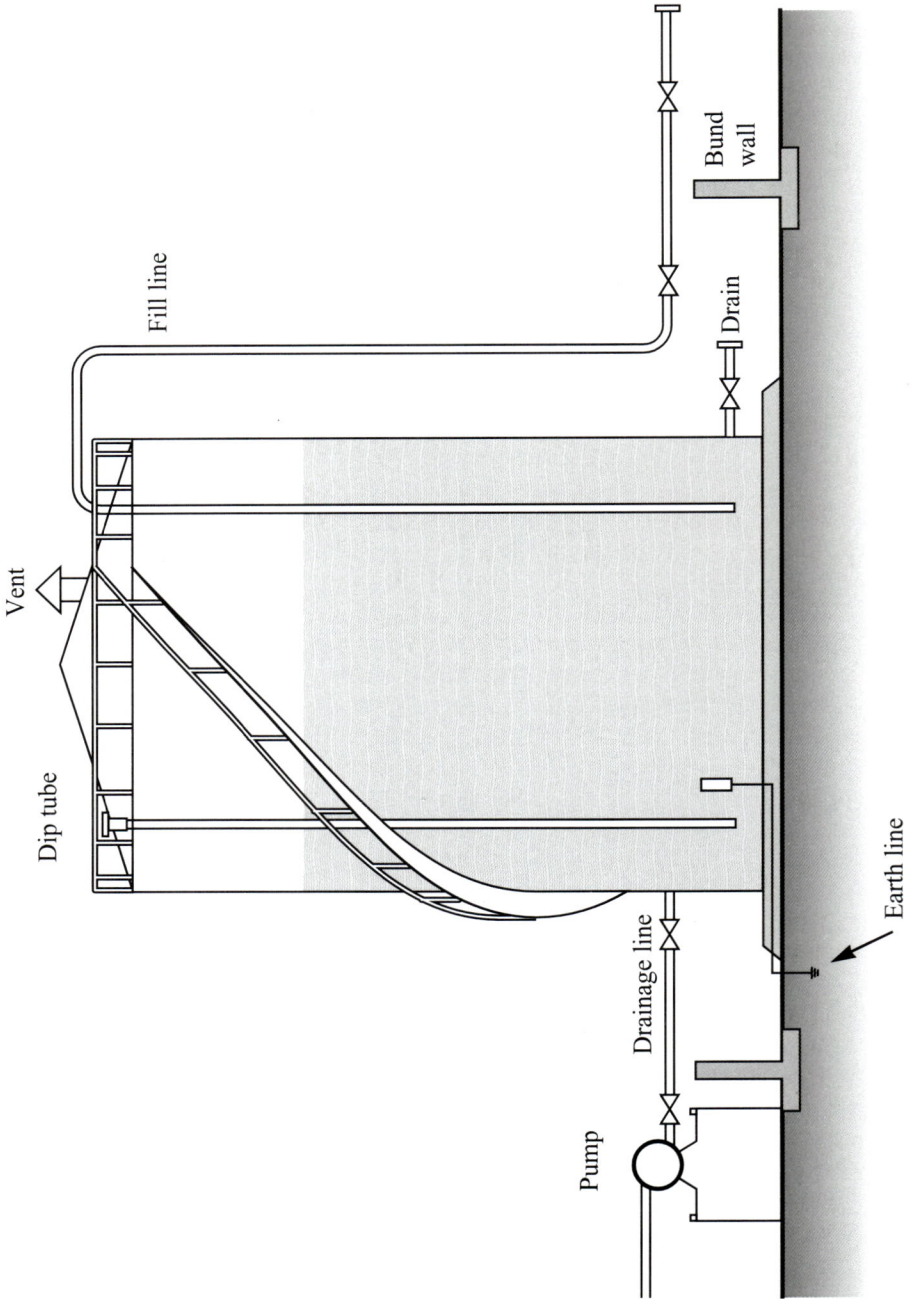

Fill line

Vent

Dip tube

Drainage line

Pump

Bund wall

Drain

Earth line

Figure 6 Typical underground tank

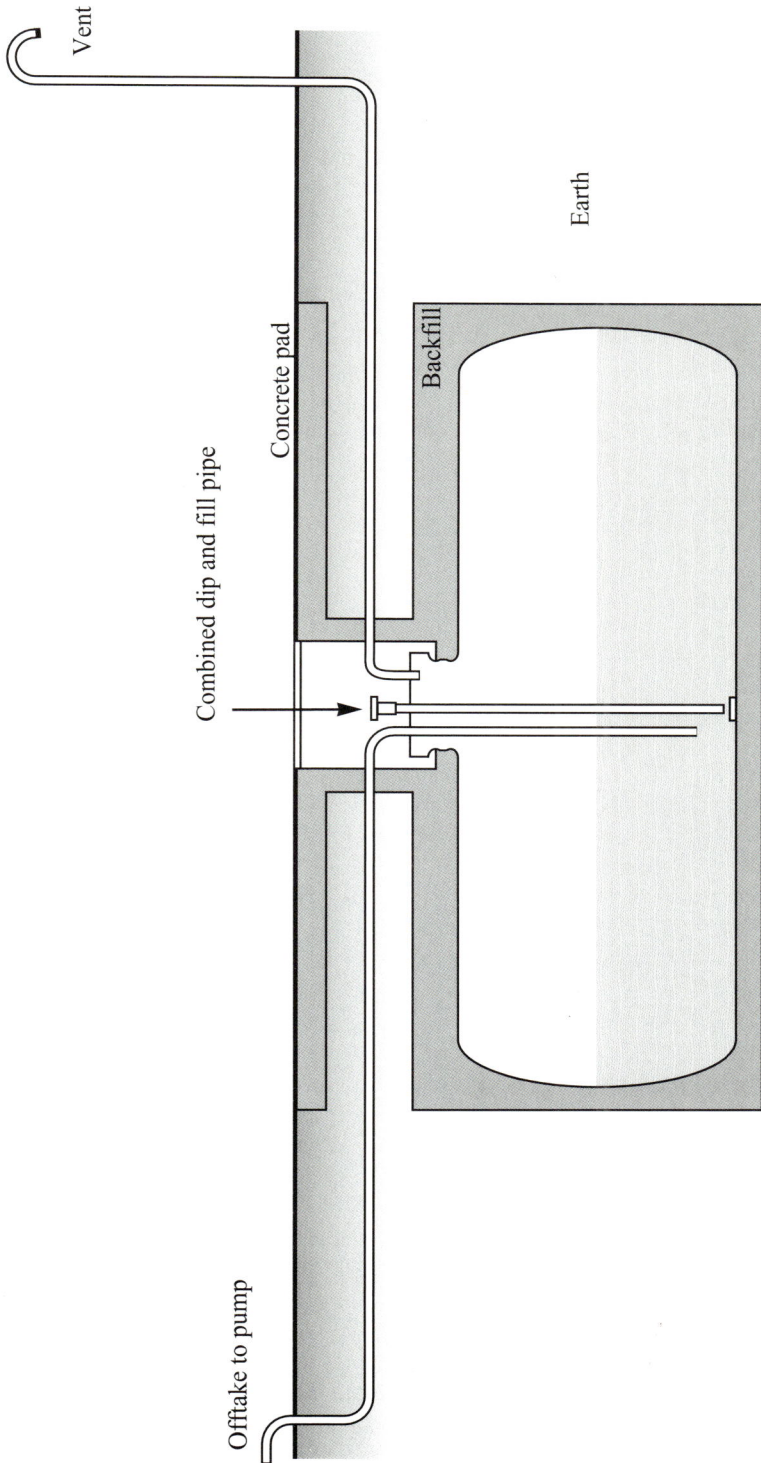

Vent

Earth

Concrete pad

Backfill

Combined dip and fill pipe

Offtake to pump

72   Internal corrosion may result from the accumulation of water in the tank. A means to remove such water may be necessary. Caution is essential when draining water from beneath the product. Reliance on a single valve to retain the tank contents is not sufficient. Two permanent in-line valves to the drainage point are recommended or temporary replacement of the blanking plate by a second valve during the draining operation.

73   Certain flammable liquids can be aggressively corrosive and may merit construction with a double tank floor. The space between the floors can be monitored, to detect failure of the tank floor.

Underlagging corrosion

74   Corrosion may occur unnoticed under thermal insulation or lagging. Underlagging corrosion should be addressed as part of the planned preventive maintenance schedule for the site.

Installing the tank

75   When installing an above-ground tank, it is important to consider the following:

- that the foundations are designed and constructed to support the full tank loading. Advice on foundations for vertical tanks is given in BS 2654[41];

- that the tank is securely anchored or weighted to avoid flotation from flood water or from spillage of liquid into the bund;

- that the supports of raised tanks are fire resistant to a two-hour standard;

- that the supports permit any movement of the tank due to temperature changes. Horizontal tanks may be supported on concrete, masonry or steel saddles. One end is secured and the other left free to move. Pipework is connected to the secure end.

76   Similarly, underground tanks require:

- foundations and adequate support (concrete or masonry);

- to be securely anchored or weighted to avoid flotation from flood water or a high water table;

- backfilling with inert material such as rounded pea gravel or with concrete. Large stones or rocks may damage the protective coating on the tank. (Note: Concrete is not suitable for double skin tanks);

- protection from loadings from above ground, particularly from traffic. A reinforced concrete slab may be suitable. Alternatively the area around the tank should be fenced off, with the perimeter of the tank clearly marked;

- an excavation of sufficient size to prevent damage to the tank's protective coating and to allow safe work during installation and backfilling.

Pipework to and from the tank

77   Pipework may be installed above or under ground. The key aims when installing pipework are:

- to ensure mechanical integrity;

- to keep the diameter and length to the minimum practicable;

- to ensure it is adequately protected from damage.

78   The reason to keep the length and diameter of pipework to a minimum is to reduce the inventory of flammable liquid in the lines. This reduces the potential for damage and spillage. There may also be economic advantages.

79   The mechanical integrity of pipework is essential. All parts of piping systems, including valve seals and flange gaskets, should be made from material compatible with the liquids being handled. They should be constructed to a suitable standard such as the American National Standards Institute Standard B31.3 *Process piping* which is supported by the *EEMUA supplement 153*[51,52].

80   Metal pipework should generally be used. Where metal pipework is not suitable such as where product purity is an issue, other materials may be used if an equivalent standard of construction can be achieved.

81   The possibility of leakage may be reduced by keeping the number of joints to a minimum and by using welded joints rather than flanged or screwed, particularly for joints underground.

82   Pressure can build up in pipework due to the thermal expansion of liquids trapped in the pipes. For example liquid may be trapped between shut-off valves. This risk should be assessed and appropriate operating procedures should be introduced to minimise the risk. Alternatively, hydrostatic relief valves may be fitted which discharge back to the tank or to a safe place such as a sump or vessel designed for the recovery or disposal of flammable liquids.

Above-ground pipework

83   Above-ground pipework, has advantages because leaks are more readily detected and any vapour produced will normally be dissipated by natural ventilation. Examinations, modifications and repairs are also easier and corrosion can be more readily identified and controlled.

84   Piping supports should be designed to suit the piping layout. (See BS 3974 *Pipe supports*[53].) The design should allow for differential movement between tanks and pipework to allow for temperature changes in heated tanks or settlement. If supports are located near tanks a two-hour standard of fire resistance is advisable.

85   Above-ground pipework and its supports may be at risk from damage particularly from vehicles. It is advisable to design the layout of the plant to minimise the risk of physical damage. Alternatively, the use of impact protection such as barriers or bollards may be appropriate.

Underground pipework

86   Underground pipework may have advantages: providing better fire protection; saving space; and providing greater security. But leakage resulting from damage or corrosion, may be difficult to detect leading to ground contamination and potential environmental problems.

87   Underground pipework should be laid in a shallow concrete or masonry-lined trench provided with load bearing covers. The design of the trench should prevent water or moisture from accumulating around the pipework and allow for inspection of the pipework, particularly joints. The design should also allow for any extra loading imposed, such as by vehicles. The route of the trench should be recorded and marked at ground level.

88   The same trench should not be used for piping carrying corrosive or reactive materials such as oxygen or chlorine. In addition, the same trench should not normally be used for electrical cables. Where this is not practicable, the cables should be selected and installed in accordance with BS 5345 *Code of practice for selection, installation and maintenance of electrical apparatus for use in potentially explosive atmospheres*[36].

Flexible hoses

89   Flexible hoses should only be used where rigid piping is unsuitable, such as at filling connections or where vibration is a problem. Hoses should be made to a standard suitable for the application and should be compatible with the materials handled. They should be adequately supported (for example by slings or saddles) so that the bend radius is not less than the minimum recommended by the manufacturer.

90   When they are not in use, flexible hoses should be protected from accidental damage, extremes of temperature and direct sunlight. They should be inspected daily for signs of leaks, wear and mechanical damage, and examined and pressure tested about once a year according to the manufacturer's recommendations. Hoses should be electrically continuous or bridged with an earthing cable to avoid electrostatic charging.

Tank connections and fittings

91   Storage tank filling and emptying connections, and openings for dipping and venting should be located at least 4 m from any source of ignition, building opening, trench or depression. Any drain in the vicinity should be either fitted with an interceptor or routed to an appropriate waste collection/treatment facility.

92   The connecting point for filling or discharge of above-ground tanks should be outside the bund wall, close to the tanker stand. This will ensure that the flexible connecting hose is kept short and will also ease access. It may be necessary to protect the tank connections to prevent mechanical damage by tanker vehicles.

93   Filling above-ground tanks from road tankers can be done either using a vehicle pump or a fixed pump on site. Use of a fixed pump has advantages as all the equipment on the vehicle can be switched off during off-loading, and the vehicle flexible hose and coupling is not subject to pump discharge pressures. Filling points should be equipped with non-return valves, close to the shut-off valve to minimise any spillage if the shut-off valve fails to seal.

94   Filling lines should be fitted with a suitable flange or coupling to connect with the hose of the delivery vehicle, rail car etc, and should be capped when not in use. A locking cap may be advisable. Spillage from making and breaking connections should be contained by a drip tray or a low sill, or be drained to a safe place. An interceptor for liquids not miscible with water, or other suitable collection method, may be required.

95   The end of the tank filling line should extend below the lowest normal operating level of the liquid, to minimise the generation of static electricity from splash filling. To prevent syphoning, the line should be self draining. Where separate lines are used for filling and emptying, a liquid seal can be maintained by ending the discharge line at least 150 mm above the bottom of the filling line. To minimise the risk of tank leakage, it is preferable for lines to enter the tank at the top. This may not always be reasonably practicable, particularly for large vertical tanks.

96   All dip rods and tubes should be earthed and where appropriate, an earthing lead for connection to a road tanker should be fitted. Reference should be made to BS 5958 *Control of undesirable static electricity Part 2*[54] for additional guidance on the control of static electricity.

97   Where several different liquids are loaded/unloaded from a common location, the labelling of pipes and fittings is advisable to prevent loading to or from the wrong tank. Additional precautions may be required if there is a possibility of mixing incompatible liquids. Methods of operating isolation and control valves should be indicated by labels or signs where necessary.

98   Tank connections to underground tanks may be located in the open air above the tank or in a chamber below ground (See Figure 6). The chamber may be closed by a watertight manhole cover or it may be raised slightly above ground level.

Valves

99   Each pipe connected to a tank is a potential source of a major leakage. Each pipeline connected to a tank should be provided with a suitable shut-off valve which is fire-safe to BS 6755 *Testing of valves: Part 2: Specification for fire type-testing requirements*[55]. The shut-off valves should be located inside the bund wall and close to the tank. The tank filling line should also be fitted with a shut-off valve outside the bund wall and close to the filling connection. Any line used only for filling and which enters the tank at the bottom should also be provided with a non-return valve.

100 Other valves may be necessary depending on process conditions, such as automatic double block and bleed systems to prevent back-flow of process materials into the storage tank or additional isolation valves to allow safe shutdown in an emergency. Important valves should be labelled to indicate their function and their method of operation, where necessary.

101 It is essential that isolating valves can be closed quickly in an emergency. Remotely operated shut-off valves (ROSOVs) may be necessary. They may be operated remotely by an electrical or pneumatic signal, or by a lever at ground level. In the event of a power failure, the controls to the ROSOVs should remain operational or the valve should fail-safe.

102 Tank drainage valves should be blanked off when not in use. Draining operations to remove accumulations of water from beneath the product should be carried out with caution, and procedures established so that reliance is not made on only one valve to retain the tank contents. This may involve the permanent fitting of two valves in line to the drainage point or temporary replacement of the blanking plate by an additional valve during the draining operation. When draining horizontal tanks the blank should be removed and a suitable length of piping attached to ensure that the liquid is drained away from the tank rather than underneath it.

103 All isolation valves should be tested periodically to ensure they are working correctly.

Pumps

104 Pumps are potential ignition sources and should be located outside the bund, on an impervious base, preferably in the open air. This will also avoid damage from fires or spillages in the bund and facilitate access for maintenance. The minimum recommended separation distance from buildings, boundaries and sources of ignition is 7.5 m for a large standard pump but can be reduced to 3 m for smaller pumps of less then 100 m^3/hr capacity (IP model code of safe practice part 15[35]).

105 Any leakage from pump seals may be contained by a low sill or drainage to a safe place.

106 Pumps may be located in a pump room, provided the room has adequate high and low level, natural or mechanical, ventilation. Interlocks should be fitted so that the pumps cannot be operated unless the ventilation is working satisfactorily. If the non-operation of a pump could cause a greater hazard than a lack of ventilation in the pump room, then a clearly audible alarm should be linked to the ventilation system.

107 Where a pump is controlled remotely, a stop control is needed at the pump itself, as well as at the control point.

Contents measurement

108 Every tank and tank compartment should have a suitable means of measuring the quantity of material stored. It should be tested and calibrated at the time of installation to ensure accuracy, and at regular intervals in line with an inspection and maintenance schedule.

Tank gauging systems

109 Automatic gauging is preferred to manual dipping as it allows determination of the quantity of liquid without opening the tank. The gauge measures parameters such as:

- height;

- mass;

- temperature;

- density; or

- pressure.

The readings are then used to determine the tank content.

110 The use of a high-level alarm is recommended, particularly if the person controlling the operation is remote from the tank or if toxic liquids are being handled. The alarm may also be arranged to stop the filling pump, unless such action could cause an additional hazard, for example, shock loading. A high, high-level trip may also be fitted, which will trigger shutdown of the pump or divert the flow, if no action has been taken following the high-level alarm. This high, high-level trip should be independent of the gauging system to provide overfill protection if the gauging system fails.

Dipping

111 Where gauging is done by dip rods, a suitable dip tube should be provided, with the dipping rod substantially smaller in diameter than the dip tube to minimise measurement errors. Dipping should not be done through open manholes.

112 Dipsticks are potential sources of ignition in that they may produce frictional heating or sparking, or static electricity. It is important that they are made of non-sparking alloys and are earthed. Reference may be made to BS 5958 *Control of undesirable static electricity Part 2*[54].

113 Manual dipping is not as accurate as an automatic gauge but provides an adequate estimate of the contents. It is important that each tank has its own calibrated dipstick, not to be used for other tanks. It may be necessary to protect the bottom of the tank to avoid damage from repeated dipping.

114 Dipsticks for large tanks are difficult to handle. Dip tapes may be an alternative. They measure depth and are used with calibration tables for individual tanks.

Vents

115 During normal tank operation, the pressure in the tank may vary. Pressures may increase during filling or if the ambient temperature rises. Conversely pressures may drop during emptying or with temperature falls. The tank venting system should provide:

- normal pressure relief;

- normal vacuum relief;

- emergency pressure relief.

116 Traditionally vents discharged into the atmosphere but there is increasing environmental pressure for vapour emission controls. Vapour recovery systems are now a legal requirement[10] for petrol storage installations and it is likely that the requirements will be extended to other flammable liquids. Further information on the design and operation of vapour recovery systems is contained in the IP *Guidelines for the design and operation of gasoline vapour emission controls*[56].

117 If flammable vapours are discharged into the open air, they may ignite if there are ignition sources nearby. The minimum recommended separation distance of vent outlets from sources of ignition, air intakes, buildings, walkways and the site boundary is 3 m. Vents should be located on top of the tank. The discharge height above the tank and above the ground should be sufficient to ensure safe dispersion of the vapours. A discharge height of 0.3 m above the tank or at least 3 m (preferably 5 m) above ground level, whichever is the higher, is usually adequate. The height of the vent outlet should be above the liquid level in the tanker. It may be necessary to increase the recommended separation distances and discharge height of the vent if

there is a possibility of poor vapour dispersion and to meet the requirements of the Environmental Protection Act.

118 Lightning or other ignition sources may ignite the vented vapours from atmospheric vents. A flame arrester installed at the vent outlet will prevent the flames spreading into the tank. A flame arrester should normally be installed at the vent outlet of a fixed-roof tank containing a liquid with a flashpoint below 21°C. Flame arresters need regular maintenance to prevent blocking by paint, scale or other material. They should be incorporated into a planned preventive inspection scheme. A flame arrester is not advisable where the liquid stored is liable to polymerise or foul the arrester. Further advice on lightning protection is given in BS 6651: 1992 *Code of practice for protection of structures against lightning*[57].

119 Pressure relief valves or vents prevent excessive pressure build-up and vacuum valves prevent the tank collapsing due to a negative pressure in the tank. These functions may be combined in a pressure-vacuum (PV) valve. PV valves are recommended (see BS 2654[41]) for use on atmospheric storage tanks in which a product with a flashpoint below 38°C is stored, and for use on tanks containing product that is heated above its flashpoint. A flame arrester is not generally considered necessary for use in conjunction with a PV valve because, even at low settings, the gas efflux velocity exceeds the flame speeds of most hydrocarbon gases.

120 It is essential that the pressure control devices are correctly sized in accordance with an appropriate code or standard such as:

- BS 2654 *Specification for manufacture of vertical steel welded non-refrigerated storage tanks with butt-welded shells for the petroleum industry*[41]; or

- API 2000 *Venting atmospheric and low-pressure storage tanks (non-refrigerated and refrigerated)*[58].

Emergency relief venting

121 The vents described above are designed to cope with the pressure fluctuations during normal operation. Additional pressure relief is necessary for above-ground tanks to cope with possible fire engulfment.

122 Emergency relief venting may be provided by:

- larger or additional vents;

- manhole or hatch covers which lift under abnormal internal pressure;

- a weak wall-to-roof joint;

- purpose-built relief devices.

123 Again, it is essential that the emergency relief devices are correctly sized in accordance with an appropriate code or standard such as BS 2654[41] or API 2000[58].

Fire protection

124 It may be necessary to provide fire protection where the storage conditions are less than ideal, such as where it is difficult to achieve adequate separation distances. Fire protection measures can be provided by:

- fire resistant claddings or coatings;

- fire walls;

- water cooling systems;

- foam blankets or extinguishing systems.

125 Combinations of the different measures may be used. Fire protection systems should be included in the inspection and maintenance schedule for the facility. Routine testing of water spray and deluge systems may be necessary. Further advice on fire protection is given in the IP *Fire precautions at petroleum refineries and bulk storage installations: model code of safe practice part 19*[37].

Fire resistant claddings or coatings

126 Fire resistant claddings or coatings may be used to protect the tank from adjacent fires or from a liquid pool fire around its base. Particular consideration should be given to the fire resistance of structures which support vessels. Collapse in a fire could escalate the incident. Fire protection of structural steel should provide a minimum protection of two hours (see BS 476 *Fire tests on building materials and structures*[59] and BS 5908 *Code of practice for fire precautions in the chemical and allied industries*[60]).

127 Thermal insulation materials are often used to reduce heat loss or heat gain. These materials may not provide fire protection unless specifically designed for the purpose.

Fire walls

128 A fire wall may be used to give additional protection to small tanks. They are not usually practicable or economic for larger tanks. Where a fire wall is installed, it should be at least the height of the tank, with a minimum height of 2 m, and should normally be sited between 1 and 3 m from the tank. It may form part of the bund wall or a building wall. A fire wall should normally be provided on only one side of a tank, to ensure adequate ventilation. The wall should be long enough to ensure that the distance between the tank and a building, boundary,

process plant or source of ignition is at least the appropriate distance in Table 2, measured around the ends of the wall.

129 To be effective a fire wall should:

- have no holes in it;

- have at least half-hour fire resistance;

- be weather-resistant;

- be sufficiently robust to withstand foreseeable accidental damage.

A reinforced concrete or masonry construction is recommended.

Water cooling systems

130 Water sprays or deluge systems are used primarily to provide cooling and so protect the tank from the damaging effects of an adjacent fire or a liquid pool fire at its base.

131 The water application rates will depend on the level of thermal radiation to which the tank and associated equipment may be exposed. The recommended rate[37] to protect a fixed-roof tank from a pool fire at its base is not less than 10 $l/min/m^2$ of exposed uninsulated surface. Protection of a tank from an adjacent fire depends on various factors such as the distance from the fire. A water rate of 2 $l/min/m^2$ is considered to be the minimum application rate for tank surfaces exposed to radiation from a non-impinging fire in adjacent equipment.

132 The application of water to the roof of floating-roof tanks is not recommended. For rim fires, water may be applied to the vertical tank walls while a foam blanket is applied to the roof.

Foam systems

133 Foam systems may be used to extinguish a fire or blanket spillages of flammable liquid and so reduce the risk of ignition. To avoid the build-up of static charges and possible ignition, foam should be applied using a foam pourer and not by jet.

Bonding and earthing

Static electricity

134 Static electricity is generated when movement separates charge which can then accumulate on plant and equipment, and on liquid surfaces. If the plant is not earthed or the liquid has a low electrical conductivity, then the charge may be generated faster than it can

dissipate. Eventually, there may be an electrical discharge or spark. If this has sufficient energy it could ignite a flammable gas or vapour.

135 To minimise the accumulation of electrostatic charge and prevent incendive sparks, all metal parts of the storage installation should be bonded together and earthed. A maximum resistance to earth of 10 ohms is recommended. It should be possible to disconnect the earthing facilities for periodic test measurement. Further advice on earthing and bonding is in BS 7430: 1991 *Code of practice for earthing*[61].

136 If the liquid has a particularly low electrical conductivity and is being stored above its flashpoint, it may be advisable to store it under a blanket of nitrogen[80] or inject it with an antistatic additive.

Bunding

137 The probability of a major leak from a well-designed and maintained storage system is low, particularly if overspill protection has been fitted. However, the consequences of a spillage of flammable liquid are potentially catastrophic. Therefore measures to contain spillages or leaks from storage tanks are essential.

138 Bunding is the method used to contain a liquid which has spilled or leaked from a vessel. It is recommended that bunding is provided for all flammable liquids with a flashpoint of 55°C or below, and for materials which are stored at temperatures above their flashpoints. The Highly Flammable Liquids and Liquefied Petroleum Gases Regulations 1972[7] require bunding for stored material with a flashpoint of 32°C and below.

139 The purpose of bunding is to:

- prevent the flammable liquid or vapour from reaching ignition sources;

- prevent the liquid entering the drainage or water systems where it may spread to uncontrolled ignition sources;

- allow the controlled recovery or treatment of the spilled material;

- minimise the surface area of the liquid and so reduce the size of any fire that may occur;

- prevent the spread of burning liquids which could present a hazard to other plant or personnel both on and off site;

- prevent contamination of land and water courses.

140 The bund should have sufficient capacity to contain the largest predictable spillage. A bund capacity of 110% of the capacity of the largest storage vessel located within the bund will normally be sufficient. When estimating the bund capacity, the space occupied by other tanks should be taken into account.

141 Smaller capacity bunds may be acceptable, where liquid can be directed to a separate evaporation area or impounding basin, using where necessary diversion walls up to 0.5 m high. A reduced capacity may also be justifiable for large tanks, in cases where there is no risk of pollution or of hazard to the public. This reduced capacity should be not less than 75% of the largest vessel located within the bund.

142 Individual bunding is to be preferred to common bunding, particularly for large tanks. Where several tanks are contained in one bunded area, intermediate lower bund walls are recommended to divide tanks into groups to contain small spillages and to minimise the surface area of any spillage. This may significantly limit the spread of fire. The total capacity of tanks in a bund should not exceed 60 000 m^3 (120 000 m^3 for floating-roof tanks).

143 The bund wall should have sufficient strength to contain any spillage or fire-fighting water. For example, a bund wall constructed of 225 mm brick or block with a height in excess of 600 mm is likely to collapse if required to contain major spillages. If a height greater than 600 mm is required then additional strengthening will be needed, such as using greater thickness of brick or block, reinforced concrete or buttresses. A fixed means of escape from the bund may be necessary.

144 The bund wall should not be constructed too close to the tank. Minimum recommended separation distances between tank and bund wall are 1 m for tanks up to 100 m^3 and 2 m for tanks above 100 m^3.

145 The design of the bund wall is a compromise between minimising the surface area of the liquid that may be spilled and minimising the height of the bund wall. Increasing the bunded area and locating lower bund walls away from the tank provides better ventilation and facilitates access for fire fighting. More space is taken but the hydrostatic loading on the wall will be less. The wall will be cheaper to design and construct.

146 The bund should be liquid tight. The integrity of the bund wall may be put at risk if pipework and other equipment are allowed to penetrate it. If it is necessary to pass pipes through the bund wall, for example to the pump, then the effect on the structural strength should be assessed. Additional measures may be needed to ensure that the bund wall remains liquid tight.

147 The floor of the bund should be of concrete or other material substantially impervious to the liquid being stored, and with drainage where necessary to prevent minor spillage collecting near tanks. Stone chippings and similar materials may be used providing the underlying

ground is impervious. A suitable buried membrane can also be used as can specially designed systems using the water table to retain liquids not miscible with water.

148 Surface water should not be allowed to collect in the bund. Sloping the bund floor from the tank will allow water to be siphoned or pumped over the bund wall. If an electrically driven pump is used, the electrical equipment should either be outside any hazardous area or be of a type suitable for the zone in which it is used.

149 Removal of surface water using pumps and siphons is not always practicable, particularly for large bunds. An alternative is to use a bund drain but if they are left open the integrity of the bund is destroyed. If a bund drain is used, there should be a system of work to ensure the valve remains closed, and preferably locked, except when water is being removed. Locating the valve outside the bund wall will ease access during normal operation and in an emergency situation.

150 Where flammable liquids not miscible with water are stored, surface water from bunds should be routed through an interceptor or separator, to prevent flammable liquids entering the main drainage system. For liquids miscible with water, special drainage systems may be required.

151 No combustible material, such as vegetation, litter or rubbish, should be allowed to accumulate in the bund, as this will increase the fire risk. Weedkiller containing sodium chlorate or other oxidising substances should not be used at storage areas or tanker stands because of the increased fire hazard. Similarly, the bund should not be used for the storage of flammable liquid containers, gas cylinders (full or empty) or other hazardous substances.

152 Bunds can be easily damaged particularly by vehicles. Damage may be prevented by using impact protection, such as crash barriers or bollards.

Marking tanks and fittings

153 A requirement of the Highly Flammable Liquids and Liquefied Petroleum Gases Regulations 1972[7] is that tanks containing highly flammable liquids should be clearly identified and marked. The marking should state 'highly flammable', or 'flashpoint below 32°C' or 'flashpoint in the range of 22°C to 32°C'. Other appropriate markings may be acceptable.

154 Where marking a tank is impracticable, the words 'Highly Flammable Liquid' should be displayed as near to the tank as is practicable. Other warning notices such as 'No Smoking' and 'No Naked Lights' may be appropriate.

155 The Health and Safety (Safety Signs and Signals) Regulations 1996[62] require safety signs to be provided where the risks to employees cannot be avoided or adequately reduced by other means. It may be necessary to provide labelling of pipes, sampling points, joints, valves, etc.

Possible examples include:

- locations where there are numerous pipes, in close proximity, conveying different dangerous substances, particularly if they have different hazardous properties;

- sampling or filling points and drain valves, particularly where they are located close to similar points for other pipes conveying dangerous substances;

- where there have been significant alterations or additions to fittings and pipe runs.

Lighting

156 Working areas associated with storage tanks, including loading and unloading points, should be adequately lit when in use. An average illuminance of at least 50 lux is recommended at ground level and on stairs, access platforms, etc. It may be necessary to increase this to 100 lux where perception of detail is required, for example to read level gauges. More detailed advice is in the book HSG38 *Lighting at work*[63].

Weather protection

157 Small above-ground tanks may be protected by a dutch-barn type structure of lightweight and generally non-combustible construction, and with at least two open sides to ensure adequate ventilation.

Testing of tanks and pipework

158 The manufacturer will normally pressure test tanks before supply in accordance with the design code used. For example, steel tanks made to BS 2594[40] receive a pressure test of 0.7 bar(g) at the tank top and a vacuum test of 10 mbar. For GRP tanks made to BS 4994[42] the pressure required will depend on the design options exercised but will normally be 1.3 x design pressure. For both types of tank, hydraulic testing is preferred to pneumatic testing for safety reasons. (For further information see Guidance Note GS4 *Safety in pressure testing*[64].)

159 Before filling with flammable liquids, leak testing of the installed tanks and pipework is required. Both steel tanks made to BS 2594 and GRP tanks made to BS 4994 should be tested to 0.5 bar(g) at the tank top. Hydraulic testing is again preferred to pneumatic, although air may be used as a means of applying pressure to water-filled tanks and piping.

160 Before using water it is important to check that all parts of the system, including pipelines and supports, are strong enough to withstand the hydraulic loading, bearing in mind any difference in specific gravity between water and the liquid to be stored in the tank. All leaks or other faults should be corrected before the tank is first used.

161 Care should be taken to ensure the compatibility of the test medium with the material of construction. For example, use of saline water in stainless steel tanks may lead to chloride corrosion cracking. After testing, the test medium should be drained and the tank dried where necessary, to prevent contamination of the stored liquid.

Heated tanks

162 Viscous liquids are often heated to ease pumping. Additional precautions are needed to ensure that the storage tank is suitable for use as a heated tank. These precautions are outlined in the following paragraphs.

163 Heated tanks and their associated heating equipment should be constructed to appropriate standards such as:

- BS 799 *Oil burning equipment Part 5 Oil storage tanks*[65];

- BS 5410 *Code of practice for oil firing*[66];

- BS 806 *Design and construction of ferrous piping installations for and in connection with land boilers*[67].

164 Locating the outlet pipe above the heating coil or element will prevent exposure of any internal heated surface or any temperature control sensor. A second drain pipe may be fitted at a lower level so that the tank can be completely emptied when necessary. This pipe should be fitted with a closed valve and a blank flange so that it cannot be used during normal operations. If this arrangement is not feasible then an alternative is to fit a low liquid level alarm linked to a heater cut-out.

Temperature control

165 The temperature of the tank should be controlled using a thermostat or similar device. It is good practice to select the minimum temperature sufficient for the purpose, preferably below the flashpoint of the liquid. Control will be easier if the heating rate is slow.

166 As well as the thermostat control, it is advisable to have an independent cut-out device which will shut down the heater completely (no automatic reset) if the temperature exceeds a set high point. This is particularly important if the flammable liquids could be heated above their flashpoint in normal operation or under fault conditions.

167 The temperature sensor (independent of the thermostat) should be located where it is continuously immersed in the liquid. A second temperature sensor may be advantageous to indicate possible problems with the thermostat.

168 It is important to maintain and recalibrate temperature probes, thermostats and associated equipment. They should be included in the preventive maintenance schedule.

169 Heaters should be used only when there is at least 150 mm of liquid covering the heating coil. The tank should not be emptied until the tubes have cooled to the temperature of the liquid. It may be advisable to install a low level alarm to ensure the heaters are not uncovered inadvertently.

170 Where vents, filters, etc are liable to become blocked, or a build-up of coke or other material is liable to occur, a regular system of inspection and cleaning is necessary. This is particularly important for vents, as blockage by, for example, polymerisation, sublimation or condensation of product, may cause damage to the tank. In some cases trace heating may be used to minimise the problem. Where electric surface heating is used, it should be selected and installed in accordance with the recommendations in BS 6351 *Electrical surface heating*[68] (in three parts).

The storage of flammable liquids in tanks

LOADING AND UNLOADING FACILITIES

171 This section provides guidance on road and rail transfer facilities. It does not cover loading and unloading from ships. If required, advice is available in the HSE Guidance Note GS40 *The loading and unloading of bulk flammable liquids and gases at harbours and inland waterways*[23].

172 All equipment including pumps, valves and hoses should be suitable for the liquids being handled and for the conditions of use. They should be made to an appropriate British Standard or equivalent. Some tankers have their own off-loading pump. If these are used, checks should be made to ensure that they are electrically protected and are of a capacity matched to the discharge pipework and the tank installation. Where vehicles are bottom loaded, the recommendations in the IP *Code of practice for road tank vehicles equipped for bottom loading and vapour recovery*[69] should be followed.

Loading and unloading of road tankers

Location

173 Loading/unloading bays for road tankers should be located in a safe, well-ventilated position. The minimum recommended distance of a filling point from occupied buildings, the site boundary and fixed sources of ignition is 10 m.

174 The loading/unloading bay should have easy access and exit for tankers, preferably without reversing. The loading/unloading area and the access road should preferably be dedicated to tanker use only. If this is not practicable, barriers to control access by other vehicles and pedestrians may be necessary during transfer operations.

175 A separate parking bay for road tankers waiting to load or unload is advisable so that vehicles and documents can be checked with minimum interference to traffic flow. Tankers should not wait on public roads or busy internal roads.

176 Level ground is desirable, surfaced with a material resistant to the liquids being handled. A small gradient may be beneficial if this assists drainage. The drainage should be designed to minimise the surface area of any spillage and lead it away from vehicles to a slop tank or interceptor.

Design of road tanker loading/unloading facility

177 To minimise the risk of overfilling, tankers should normally be loaded using a flow meter with a trip to stop the pump and close a shut-off valve automatically when a pre-set quantity has been delivered. Use of an independent high-level or overflow alarm is recommended to provide a warning if the meter fails. Meters may be protected by installing flow control valves.

178 Before liquids are unloaded from tankers into storage tanks, particular attention should be paid to ensuring enough ullage space is available in the storage tank to receive the load. The use of high-level alarms on storage tanks is described in paragraph 110. To reduce the likelihood of spillage, the use of self-sealing couplings on the hose connections should be considered.

179 Precautions should be taken against spillage due to vehicles being moved with the hoses still connected or arms still in place. This can be done by providing barriers across the tanker stance, brake interlocks on the vehicle or breakaway couplings on the hose connections.

180 In addition to any automatic shut-off devices on the tanker or the tank, an emergency stop button should be installed at the loading/unloading point which will activate a quick-action shut-off valve or pump stop control. This will enable the operator/driver to stop immediately loading/unloading if a problem is observed.

181 Precautions against static electricity should be provided. These include an earthing connection for the vehicle, electrically conducting hoses and elimination of splash filling. For additional protection an interlock may be fitted to prevent operation of the control valve or loading pump until the earth connection is made (see also BS 5958 Part 2[54]). Splash filling may be avoided by ensuring that the fill pipe in a top loading operation reaches to the bottom of the tank or tanker.

182 Safe access to equipment and safe means of escape for work above ground level is necessary. For top loading of vehicles, access gantries with stairs or ladders and protective handrails will usually be required. Gantries should be made of fire-resisting materials and where necessary should include means of access to the top of the tanker vehicles.

183 Fire protection measures should be designed to minimise the risk of fire spread. This may be achieved by ensuring that a ready supply of water and/or foam is available from fixed or mobile equipment. Hand extinguishers should also be located at appropriate points within the transfer area. The loading/unloading facilities should also be fitted with easily accessible fire alarm activation points.

184 The information on tank connections and fittings, and contents measurement (paragraphs 91-114) is also relevant.

Transfer by rail

185 Most of the advice given above for road transfer can be applied to rail. In addition, the following advice is recommended for rail transfers:

- a separation distance of at least 15 m from any railway line in regular use;

- straight and level tracks with a maximum gradient of no more than 1 in 400, any dead end to slope down towards the buffers;

- isolation from other rail traffic by closing and locking barriers or points. If the siding is part of an electrified track system the siding should be electrically isolated from the rest of the system and bonded to the site main earth;

- precautions to prevent the train from moving during loading or unloading;

- precautions to prevent the locomotive acting as a source of ignition. These may include keeping a separation distance of at least 9 m between the filling hose and the locomotive unless it is protected to zone 2 standard;

- remote pump controls at intervals along the siding;

- quick action manually-operated stop valves and non-return valves on the individual lines from a common header pipe used to fill/unload two or more rail cars simultaneously. This will prevent back-feeding;

- maintenance of track and the line-side equipment to an appropriate standard.

Operation of road and rail facilities

186 All operations should be under the control of an authorised person, who should be present at all times during the transfer. In some circumstances, the authorised person may be the driver. This is common practice for the delivery of petrol in accordance with Schedule 12 of the Carriage of Dangerous Goods by Road Regulations 1996[70-75]. Before any transfer is made between a road or rail tanker and a storage installation, an authorised site representative should be notified.

187 To minimise the generation of static electricity, splash filling should be avoided, for example, by ensuring that the open end of the fill pipe is not above the normal minimum surface level of the tank contents. Part 2 of BS 5958[54] recommends that for liquids with conductivities up to 50 pS/m the inlet velocity should not exceed 1 m/s until the inlet is

covered. Subsequent flow velocities of up to 7 m/s have shown no evidence of being a hazard, providing no immiscible phase is present.

188 Static charging can also be minimised during road and rail loading by avoiding switch loading. This is a practice in which a tanker that has contained low-flashpoint liquid, such as petrol, is subsequently loaded with a higher-flashpoint liquid, such as kerosene.

189 Written instructions should be provided covering all aspects of the operation. These may include:

- the careful checking of load details and tank ullages;

- inspection of hoses and other items of equipment;

- the measures to prevent the vehicle moving while hoses are connected;

- tanker earthing;

- the transfer procedure; and

- emergency procedures.

190 Before unloading the tanker, placards and the accompanying delivery notes should be checked to ensure, so far as is reasonably practicable, that the material being delivered is what it is supposed to be. This is particularly important if incompatible materials are stored on site. Even substituting a flammable liquid with a highly flammable liquid can ultimately have serious consequences, such as loading petrol into a diesel tank. Similarly, before a loaded tanker leaves site, placards and paperwork should be checked to ensure they match the load.

191 An effective means of communication should be provided between personnel involved in the loading/unloading operations, and other parts of the site such as the control room. If radios are needed they should be suitable for use in hazardous areas.

INSPECTION AND MAINTENANCE

192 Health and safety law[4,5,6,76] requires that plant and equipment is maintained in a safe condition. Storage tanks and all associated equipment, including walls and fences, should be properly maintained. Only personnel who are suitably qualified and authorised, and who fully understand the hazards, should carry out inspection and maintenance.

193 It is good practice to list the component parts of the installation on a preventive maintenance schedule, containing details of the scope and frequency of planned inspection and maintenance work. Attention should also be paid to periodic inspection of electrical equipment and operation of isolation valves. There should be regular inspection and cleaning of interceptors, bunds, vents, slop tanks, loading and unloading facilities, and any buildings where flammable vapour may be present. Fire-fighting equipment should be regularly maintained and, where appropriate, tested.

194 Examination of tanks, pipework and fittings should be carried out by a competent person. This could be a specialist inspection engineer employed by an insurance company or an employee with the appropriate qualifications and experience. A written scheme of examination should be agreed between the user and the competent person, to include the scope and frequency of thorough examination. Intervals between internal examinations should be determined using a risk assessment approach based on tank service, maintenance history and known corrosion rates. Intermediate external examinations should also be carried out on above-ground tanks. Records should be kept of all examinations, tests, modifications and major maintenance. Schemes of examination should be in writing and should be reviewed regularly. Hoses normally need to be examined and pressure-tested at least annually, and visually inspected on every day they are used.

Floating-roof tanks

195 For tanks with a floating or internal floating cover, attention should be paid to avoiding fouling or obstruction of tank connections, and to providing adequate buoyancy of the roof or cover, adequate roof space ventilation and adequate electrical bonding.

196 Regular inspection for cracks and damage to the rim seal is advisable. The drainage system may need regular attention to prevent accumulation of rainwater.

197 A safe system of work for access to the roof is also important, particularly when it is more than 2 m below the tank top, due to the possible accumulation of vapour. The system of work should include emergency procedures and means of escape, in the event of fire.

Permit-to-work systems

198 Many accidents have occurred while storage installations were being maintained, modified or demolished. The main cause is the introduction of a source of ignition, such as a cutting torch or an unprotected light, to pieces of equipment where flammable vapours remain. It is essential that any work carried out on equipment which may contain a flammable liquid or vapour is covered by a permit-to-work or similar system of authorisation. Permit procedures are described fully in *Guidance on permit-to-work systems in the petroleum industry*[77]. A typical permit will specify:

- the area to which the permit applies;

- the work to be done and the method to be used;

- the time limit on the permit;

- the precautions to ensure that all flammable materials have been removed and cannot be accidentally reintroduced.

199 Care should be taken to ensure that contractors and subcontractors are also covered by the permit or authorisation system.

Modifying the storage installation

200 Modifications may affect the mechanical or electrical integrity of the storage installation. A risk assessment should be carried out at the planning stage to identify any additional hazards that the modification may introduce. The use of a competent person to oversee the work will ensure the installation remains fit for purpose. Additional testing may be required.

Decommissioning tanks

201 Tanks which are to be taken out of use should be made safe. The method will vary with the location of the tank, the product it has contained and whether it is to be taken out of use permanently or temporarily. A risk assessment should be carried out at the planning stage to identify any additional hazards that decommissioning may introduce. The work should also be covered by a permit-to-work or similar authorisation procedure.

202 The preliminary steps in the decommissioning process (which apply also to pipework) are:

- isolation of the tank from any process, plant or storage vessel by either removing pipe sections or fitting spade pieces. Shut-off valves by themselves are not adequate;

- emptying the tank as much as possible;

- opening manholes to assist venting.

203 Tanks which are being decommissioned permanently should be made safe by thorough cleaning and gas freeing. Guidance is available in the HSE Guidance Note CS15 *The cleaning and gas freeing of tanks containing flammable residues*[78].

204 Tanks that are being decommissioned temporarily should be made safe by thorough cleaning as above, or by filling with water or an inert gas such as nitrogen. The advice given in CS15 is applicable in this situation. If inert gas is used, the tank should be labelled to make it clear that it contains a gas which could cause suffocation if the tank is entered. See also the HSE publication L101 *Safe work in confined spaces*[81]. Regular inspection will be needed to ensure that the tank remains in a safe condition.

205 Advice on the decommissioning of underground tanks is given in APEA/IP *Code of practice for the design, construction and operation of petrol filling stations*[82].

Demolishing tanks

206 Demolition of tanks which have contained flammable liquids is potentially very hazardous. Hot work can cause an explosion if undertaken before the tank and pipework has been drained and cleaned. Tanks that have contained flammable liquids need special preparation to remove flammable vapours, or associated liquids and sludges. Residues that can evolve flammable vapours when heated may be present on the walls and underside of the roof. It may be advisable to use a specialist tank demolition company with the relevant expertise and equipment.

207 Guidance is available in CS15 *The cleaning and gas freeing of tanks containing flammable residues*[78], IP *Tank cleaning safety code: model code of practice part 16*[79] and BS 6187 *Code of practice for demolition*[83].

54   *The storage of flammable liquids in tanks*

FIRE PRECAUTIONS

208 The likelihood of a major fire may be minimised by:

- good plant design and layout;

- sound engineering;

- good operating practice;

- tight control of non-routine operations such as repairs and modifications;

- instruction and training of personnel in routine operations and in emergency procedures.

209 Plant design and layout should include consideration of:

- water supplies;

- fire-protection equipment;

- fire fighting;

- means of escape;

- means of access for fire brigade appliances;

- arrangements to ensure an early call-out of the fire brigade in the event of fire;

- ability of the drainage/interceptor facilities to cope with fire water.

210 The fire authority should be consulted on these matters (at the planning stage in the case of new or altered facilities). Further guidance is available in the IP *Fire precautions at petroleum refineries and bulk storage installations: model code of safe practice part 19*[37].

Fire-fighting equipment and facilities

211 Under the Fire Service Act 1947[84] it is the responsibility of the local fire authority to make provision for fire-fighting, and to equip and maintain a fire brigade to meet normal requirements. The fire authority may make arrangements with works' fire teams to provide assistance but the local authority brigade will assume control of fire-fighting operations on arrival at a fire. It may be possible to negotiate additional assistance with nearby sites, perhaps by a mutual aid agreement.

212 The fire-fighting equipment for bulk storage of flammable liquids will depend on the quantity and type of liquid, and on the conditions of storage. Fire-fighting equipment should be provided at readily accessible locations at the storage area, including identifiable danger points such as pump rafts, hose pits and loading gantries. Protection against the weather, particularly freezing, may be required.

213 Dry powder or foam fire extinguishers (hand-held or trolley-mounted) are suitable to deal with fires from small leaks of flammable liquid. CO_2 extinguishers should be used for electrical fires. To guard against equipment failure, it is preferable to have extinguishers grouped in pairs. Fire extinguishers should be regularly inspected and tested by a competent agency.

214 For other fires that might affect the storage, eg those involving rubbish or vegetation, water hoses are appropriate. Hoses may be in reels permanently connected to a water supply, or in lengths for connection to a hydrant, and should cover all parts of the storage installation. BS 5306 *Fire extinguishing installations and equipment on premises*[85] gives advice on suitable types of equipment.

215 Facilities to deal with larger fires include an adequate water supply for fire brigade use. This may consist of hydrants, ponds, canals, etc and should be readily accessible and normally no more than 100 m from the tanks. The need for foam and the means of application may be discussed with the fire authority, taking into account the number, size, type, location and contents of tanks.

216 An adequate supply of water will also be needed to provide cooling for tanks exposed to heat from a nearby fire. The recommended rate is not less than 10 litres/m^2/min over the surface of the tank for 30 minutes. It is important that the entire tank is covered with water to prevent hotspots developing. Fixed water sprays or portable monitors are an advantage, but are normally required only where the storage conditions are less than ideal, such as where it is difficult to achieve adequate separation distances.

217 Fire water run-off may place a major strain on normal drainage facilities. Interceptors or special draining systems may be necessary, particularly at large installations, to minimise the risk of contamination of local watercourses. Consultation with the water authority, the Environment Agency and the fire authority may be appropriate.

EMERGENCY PROCEDURES

218 The impact of an incident involving flammable liquids may be drastically reduced if prompt emergency action is taken. Everyone should know what to do in the event of spills, leaks or fires involving flammable liquids. Practical training and written procedures should be provided covering:

- raising the alarm;

- calling the fire brigade;

- controlling the spill or leak;

- tackling the fire (when it is safe to do so); and

- evacuating the area safely.

219 Where an incident may affect people or property beyond the site boundary, the emergency services should be consulted. At installations subject to regulations 7-12 of the CIMAH Regulations[31], formal on-site and off-site emergency plans are required.

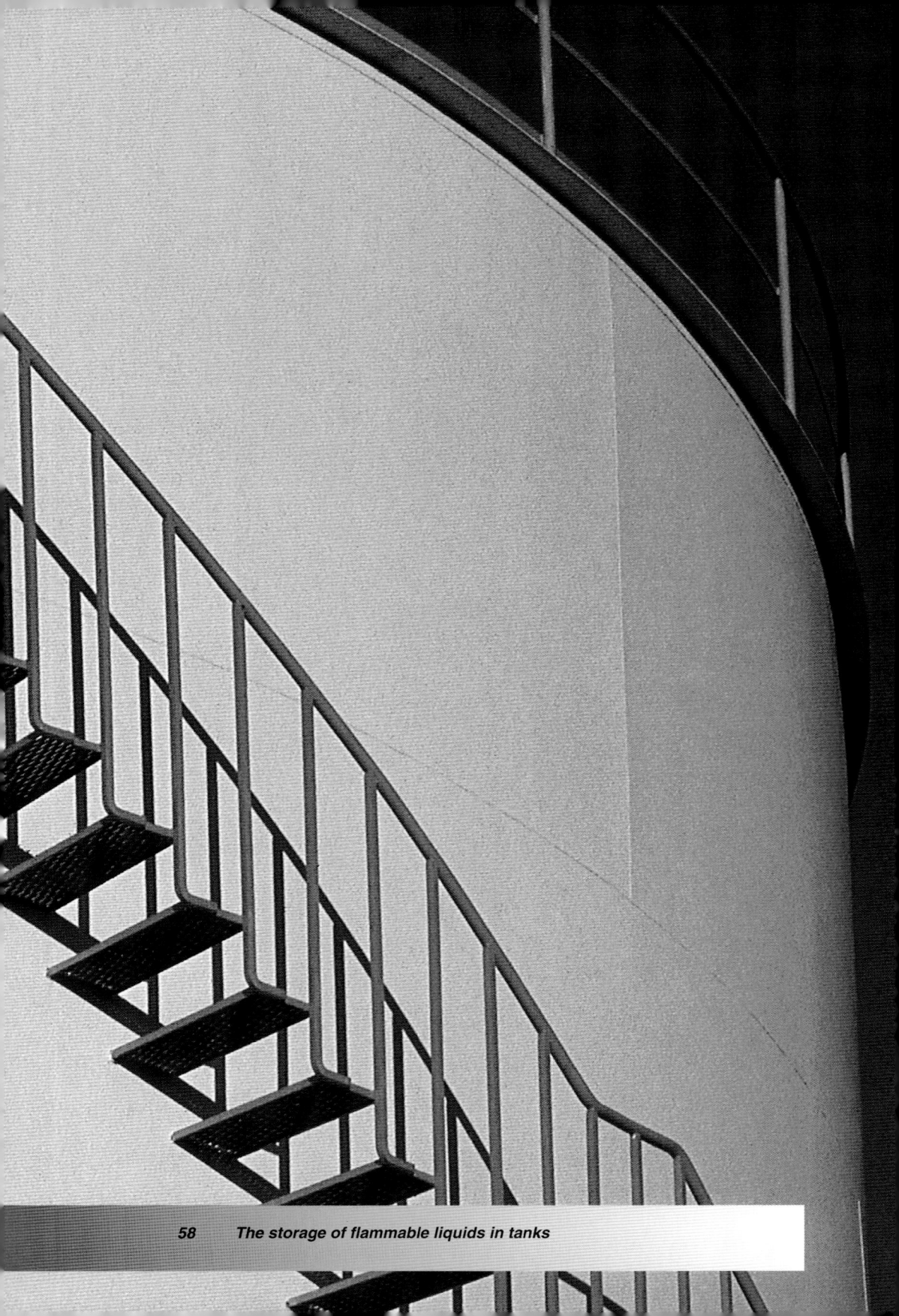

The storage of flammable liquids in tanks

SECURITY

220 The consequences of trespassing or tampering may be very serious. Good security is essential. If the storage facility is within the security area of the premises as a whole then this may give adequate protection. Otherwise, it is advisable to enclose storage areas and areas used for loading or unloading tankers by using a substantial fence at least 1.8 m high. Use of welded mesh or chain link fencing which will not obstruct ventilation is preferred.

221 For means of escape, at least two separate exits will normally be needed. One exit may be sufficient if the distance from any part of the storage area to the exit is not more than 24 m, measured around the tanks and any other obstructions. Exits should open outwards and be easily opened from inside when the area is occupied. They should be kept locked when the area is unoccupied, with access to the keys restricted to authorised personnel. A written procedure covering key control may be advisable.

The storage of flammable liquids in tanks

TRAINING

222 The provision of adequate information and training is a requirement of several pieces of legislation[1,4,76]. Everyone on site should be informed of the hazards from flammable liquids stored there and of the need to exclude sources of ignition and heat. Those handling flammable liquids should also receive specific training in both normal operating procedures and emergency procedures. Periodic retraining will usually be necessary. A typical training schedule will include the following:

- hazards and properties of the liquids being stored;

- safe operating procedures for the installation and its associated equipment;

- the purpose of the safety features, including the importance of not removing or tampering with them;

- the action to be taken if a fault in the equipment is detected;

- dealing with minor leaks and spills;

- the importance of good housekeeping and preventive maintenance;

- emergency procedures.

HIGHER-FLASHPOINT LIQUIDS

223 For liquids with a flashpoint in the range of 32-55°C some of the precautions described in this book may not be necessary. These liquids will not normally produce a flammable atmosphere unless they are stored at temperatures above their flashpoint.

224 The following paragraphs indicate where the advice in the proceeding guidance may be relaxed for higher-flashpoint liquids stored at temperatures below their flashpoint. If no variation is shown for any particular aspect, the standards in the main text apply.

Sources of ignition

225 Where the temperature of a liquid is not likely to be raised above its flashpoint, and there is little likelihood of a flammable mist or spray occurring, the liquid may be considered not to give rise to a hazardous area. Protection of nearby electrical equipment is not then required. It is important however that there should be no likelihood of local heating of the liquid, which might produce a flammable vapour.

226 For tanks containing higher-flashpoint liquids at temperatures above their flashpoint, electrical equipment within 1m of tank vents and other openings should be protected to zone 2 standards. Equipment located in the vapour space inside such tanks should be to zone 0 standards.

227 Irrespective of storage temperature, installations where liquid can escape as a mist or spray may require explosion-protection of adjacent electrical equipment. An example is a pump used to fill or empty a tank.

228 In all cases precautions against the introduction of other sources of ignition such as smoking and hot work will be needed.

229 Protection against vehicles acting as a source of ignition is not required for vehicles used or parked in storage areas containing only higher-flashpoint liquids.

Location of tanks above ground

230 In Table 2 the separation distance from buildings etc, for tanks above 250 m^3 capacity may be reduced to 10 m.

231 The recommended minimum separation distances for a tank containing higher-flashpoint liquid are:

- from another tank containing a higher-flashpoint liquid: the minimum needed for safe construction and operation;

- from a tank containing a low flashpoint liquid: in accordance with Table 3.

Storage in buildings

232 It is advisable to store all classes of flammable liquids outside wherever reasonably practicable. Where higher-flashpoint liquids are stored in buildings the precautions in paragraphs 56-59 are relevant, with the following changes:

- a lightweight roof is recommended but other protection against explosion is not required;

- a lower standard of ventilation, eg a limited number of air bricks in external walls, is adequate;

- the building need not be single-storey (but the tanks should be located on the ground floor); and

- a fixed water installation is not necessary.

Venting

233 The minimum recommended heights for vent outlets do not apply to higher-flashpoint liquids. The separation distance from buildings, etc may be reduced to 1 m. Flame arresters are not required but fire engulfment relief should be provided.

Marking and labelling

234 Tanks should be marked 'Flammable Liquid'.

Road and rail tankers

235 The recommended separation distance between road transfer facilities and buildings etc may be reduced to 5 m. The restriction on approach of locomotives need not be applied.

APPENDIX 1
LEGAL
REQUIREMENTS

Management of Health and Safety at Work Regulations 1996

1   Under these Regulations[1] every employer has a duty to carry out an assessment of the risks to the health and safety of employees, and of anyone who may be affected by the work activity. This is so that hazards may be identified and the appropriate preventive and protective measures introduced.

2   An Approved Code of Practice *Management of health and safety at work*[2] gives guidance on the provisions of these Regulations. An HSE leaflet *5 steps to risk assessment*[3] gives simple general advice on the steps involved in the risk assessment process.

Health and Safety At Work etc Act 1974

3   The Health and Safety at Work etc Act 1974[4] (HSW) requires employers to provide and maintain safe systems of work. They are also required to take all reasonable precautions to ensure the health and safety of employees, and of anybody else who could be affected by the work activity. Employers and the self-employed also have a legal duty to take care of their own and other people's health and safety.

4   The HSW Act is enforced either by HSE or by local authorities, as determined by the Health and Safety (Enforcing Authority) Regulations 1989[6]. Further advice on these matters is obtainable from local area offices of HSE or the environmental health department of the local authority, as appropriate. Guidance on the Act is also available in an HSE booklet *A guide to the Health and Safety at Work etc Act 1974*[5].

Highly Flammable Liquids and Liquefied Petroleum Gases Regulations 1972

5   These Regulations[7] (sometimes known as the HFL Regulations) apply when liquids with a flashpoint of less than 32°C, and which support combustion (when tested in the prescribed manner), are present at premises subject to the Factories Act 1961[93].

6   The Regulations require that precautions should be taken to reduce the risk of fires and explosions, where flammable liquids or gases are stored or processed. These precautions include measures to prevent and manage leaks, spills and dangerous concentrations of vapours and to control ignition sources.

7   An exception to the storage requirements of these Regulations applies where a petroleum licence is in force. This exception is likely to be removed by new petroleum Regulations which are currently in preparation. Under the new Regulations, petroleum stored at workplaces will also be subject to the HFL Regulations.

The Provision and Use of Work Equipment Regulations 1992

8   The aim of these Regulations (known as the PUWER Regulations) is to ensure that safe work equipment is provided and is safely used. Under these Regulations[76] employers must ensure that:

- suitable equipment is provided for the work involved;

- information and instruction are adequate;

- equipment is maintained in good working order and repair;

- training is provided for operators and supervisors;

- equipment is safeguarded to prevent risks from mechanical and other specific hazards;

- equipment is provided with appropriate and effective controls;

- maintenance is carried out safely.

9   Regulation 12 is particularly relevant to equipment associated with flammable liquids. It requires employers to ensure that people using work equipment are not exposed to hazards arising from:

- equipment catching fire or overheating;

- the unintended or premature discharge of any liquid or vapour;

- the unintended or premature explosion of the work equipment or any substance used or stored in it.

10   The Regulations are currently under revision. The new Regulations (PUWER 2) are expected to come into force in late 1998.

The Petroleum (Consolidation) Act 1928

11   The Act[14] defines petroleum and petroleum spirit, and it requires the keeping of such liquids (except for small specified quantities) to be authorised by a licence, and to be in accordance with any conditions of the licence. The Petroleum (Mixtures) Order 1929[15] extends these requirements to petroleum mixtures which are defined in the Order.

12   It is expected that this Act will be repealed and replaced by new petroleum Regulations in 1998 or 1999. Petroleum stored at workplaces will be subject to the Highly Flammable Liquids and Liquefied Petroleum Gases Regulations 1972[7].

The Equipment and Protective Systems Intended for Use in Potentially Explosive Atmospheres Regulations 1996

13   These Regulations[94] describe measures to prevent ignition by equipment, and apply both to electrical and non-electrical equipment and protective systems. They apply to all equipment intended for use in potentially explosive atmospheres. The Regulations apply to all new equipment, with a transition period up to 2003. The Regulations define different categories of equipment for use in hazardous areas. The different categories of equipment cater for the different risks in zones 0, 1 and 2. Harmonised standards describe detailed methods of complying with the essential safety requirements for equipment. When equipment designed to comply with the Regulations becomes available it will carry the CE mark and the Ex (in a hexagon) mark.

Factories Act 1961

14   This Act[93] defines a 'factory' and contains many general and detailed provisions relating to work activities in factories. Section 31(3) contains specific requirements relating to the opening of plant that contains any explosive or flammable gas or vapour under pressure. Section 31(4) contains specific requirements relating to the application of heat to plant that has contained any explosive or flammable substance.

Chemicals (Hazard Information and Packaging for Supply) Regulations 1994

15   These Regulations[16] are commonly referred to as CHIP. They contain requirements for the supply of chemicals. The Regulations require the supplier of chemicals to:

- classify them, that is identify their hazards;

- give information about the hazards to the people they supply, both in the form of labels and safety data sheets;

- package the chemicals safely.

16   Classifying chemicals according to the CHIP Regulations requires knowledge of physical and chemical properties, including the flashpoints of liquids, and of health and environmental effects. Chemicals are grouped into three categories of danger, according to their flashpoints:

- extremely flammable - liquids with a flashpoint lower than 0°C and a boiling point lower than or equal to 55°C;

- highly flammable - liquids with a flashpoint below 21°C but which are not extremely flammable;

- flammable - liquids with a flashpoint equal to or greater than 21°C and less than or equal to 55°C and which support combustion when tested in the prescribed manner at 55°C.

17   Flammable, highly flammable and extremely flammable liquids are all included in the scope of this guidance book. The Regulations are supported by an Approved Supply List[18] containing agreed classifications for some common substances, an approved classification and labelling guide[19], an Approved Code of Practice on safety data sheets[17] and by the guidance publication *CHIP for everyone*[20].

The Carriage of Dangerous Goods (Classification, Packaging and Labelling) and Use of Transportable Pressure Receptacles Regulations 1996

18   These Regulations[73] apply to the carriage of dangerous goods by road and rail. Their aim is to reduce the hazards involved in transporting such substances by requiring them to be correctly classified, and packaged and labelled according to that classification. They specify that dangerous substances should be carried in suitable containers which will not leak under normal handling. These should bear appropriate warning labels giving information on the nature of the hazards.

19   Two associated documents, the *Approved carriage list*[71] and the *Approved requirements and test methods for the classification and packaging of dangerous goods for carriage*[72] provide assistance to enable compliance with these Regulations. Flammable liquids classified as dangerous substances by these Regulations are those liquids which have a flashpoint of 61°C or below (with certain exceptions based on their combustibility), or liquids with a flashpoint above 61°C carried at temperatures above their flashpoint.

The Carriage of Dangerous Goods by Road Regulations 1996

20   These Regulations[70] complement the Carriage of Dangerous Goods (Classification, Packaging and Labelling) and Use of Transportable Pressure Receptacles Regulations 1996[71]. Their provisions include requirements for:

- the construction of vehicles;

- information to be received by operators and to be given to drivers;

- the marking of vehicles;

- the loading, stowage and unloading of consignments.

Electricity at Work Regulations 1989

21   These Regulations[95] impose requirements for electrical systems and equipment, including work activities on or near electrical equipment. They also require electrical equipment which is exposed to any flammable or explosive substance, including flammable liquids or vapours, to be constructed or protected so as to prevent danger.

Control of Industrial Major Accident Hazards Regulations 1984 as amended 1989/90

22   These Regulations[31] apply at two levels to certain premises where specified quantities of particular substances are stored or used, such as flammable liquids with a flashpoint below 21°C and a boiling point (at normal pressure) above 20°C. The main aim of these Regulations is to prevent major accidents occurring; a secondary objective is to limit the effects of any which do happen. A major accident is a major emission, fire or explosion resulting from uncontrolled developments which leads to serious danger to people or the environment.

23   The first level requirements apply at premises where 5000 tonnes or more of flammable liquids, as defined previously, are involved in certain industrial activities, including processing operations and storage. The second level requirements apply where 50 000 tonnes or more of flammable liquids are involved. The general requirements apply at both levels, and require the person in control of the industrial activity to demonstrate that the major accident hazards have been identified and that the activity is being operated safely. The additional requirements that apply at the second level include the submission of a written safety report, preparation of an on-site emergency plan and provision of certain information for the public. The HSE publication HSR21[32] gives guidance on these Regulations.

Control of Major Accident Hazards Involving Dangerous Substances (COMAH) Regulations

24   The COMAH Regulations are expected to replace the existing CIMAH Regulations in February 1999. The Regulations cannot be written until the text of the European Seveso II Directive is finalised.

Notification of Installations Handling Hazardous Substances Regulations (NIHHS) 1982

25   These Regulations[97] require premises with specified quantities of particular substances, such as 10 000 tonnes or more of flammable liquids with a flashpoint of less than 21°C to be notified to HSE. Following the Planning (Hazardous Substances) Act 1990 and the Planning (Hazardous Substances) Regulations 1992[98], the presence of NIHHS Schedule 1 substances and quantities, together with some from CIMAH Schedule 3[31], on, over, or under land requires consent from hazardous substances authorities. Similar provisions also apply in Scotland.

Control of Substances Hazardous to Health Regulations 1994

26   These Regulations[28] require employers to assess the risks arising from hazardous substances at work and to decide on the measures needed to protect the health of employees. The employer is also required to take appropriate action to prevent or adequately control exposure to the hazardous substance.

27   Substances covered by the Regulations include carcinogenic substances and those which, under the Chemicals (Hazard Information and Packaging for Supply) Regulations 1994[16], are labelled as very toxic, toxic, harmful, corrosive or irritant. The Regulations also cover dusts, where present in substantial quantities, and those substances assigned occupational exposure limits. Flammable liquids normally have toxic or harmful properties which bring them within the scope of these Regulations.

Health and Safety (Safety Signs and Signals) Regulations 1996

28   These Regulations[62] require the provision, maintenance and use of signs when a risk assessment has indicated the need for a sign to warn of a hazard that cannot be prevented or controlled effectively by other means.

Fire Precautions Act 1971

29   This Act[86] controls what have become known as the 'general fire precautions', covering the means of escape in case of fire, the means for ensuring the escape routes can be used safely and effectively, the means for fighting fires, the means for giving warning in the case of fire, and the training of staff in fire safety.

30   The Act allows the presence of flammable liquids to be taken into account when considering general fire precautions. The Act is enforced by the fire authorities and further guidance can be found in the Home Office publication *Guide to fire precautions in existing places of work that require a fire certificate - factories, offices, shops and railway premises*[87]. Premises without a fire certificate will be subject to the Fire Precautions (Workplace) Regulations which are scheduled to come into force in December 1997. Supporting guidance will be published in due course.

Fire Certificate (Special Premises) Regulations 1976

31   These Regulations[88] apply at premises where certain quantities of hazardous materials are processed, used or stored. For flammable liquids they apply at premises where there is a total of more than 4000 tonnes of any highly flammable liquid (as defined by the Highly Flammable Liquids and Liquefied Petroleum Gases Regulations 1972[7]), or more than 50 tonnes of any highly flammable liquid held under pressure greater than atmospheric pressure and at a temperature above its boiling point. Where these Regulations apply they take the place of the Fire Precautions Act 1971[86] and designated HSE as the enforcing authority for matters relating to general fire precautions.

Dangerous Substances (Notification and Marking of Sites) Regulations 1990

32   The purpose of these Regulations[99] is to assist the fire-fighting services by the provision of advance and on-site information on sites containing large quantities of dangerous substances. The Regulations apply at sites containing total quantities of 25 tonnes or more of dangerous substances. Dangerous substances include flammable liquids with a flashpoint below 55°C as defined by this guidance document. The Regulations require suitable signs to be erected at access points and at any locations specified by an inspector, and notification to the appropriate fire and enforcing authorities of the presence of any dangerous substances. The HSE publication HSR29[100] gives further guidance.

Reporting of Injuries, Diseases and Dangerous Occurrences Regulations (RIDDOR) 1995

33   RIDDOR[101] requires the reporting of work-related accidents, diseases and dangerous occurrences. The full list of reportable injuries, diseases and dangerous occurrences can be found in the Regulations and in the guide to the Regulations. Dangerous occurrences which are relevant to this guidance include:

- explosion, collapse or bursting of any closed vessel or associated pipework;

- a road tanker carrying a dangerous substance overturns, suffers serious damage, catches fire or the substance is released;

- explosion or fire causing suspension of normal work for over 24 hours;

- sudden uncontrolled release in a building of:
    - 100 kg or more of flammable liquid;
    - 10 kg of flammable liquid above its boiling point;
    - 10 kg or more of flammable gas; or
    - 500 kg of these substances if the release is in the open air;

- accidental release of any substance which may damage health.

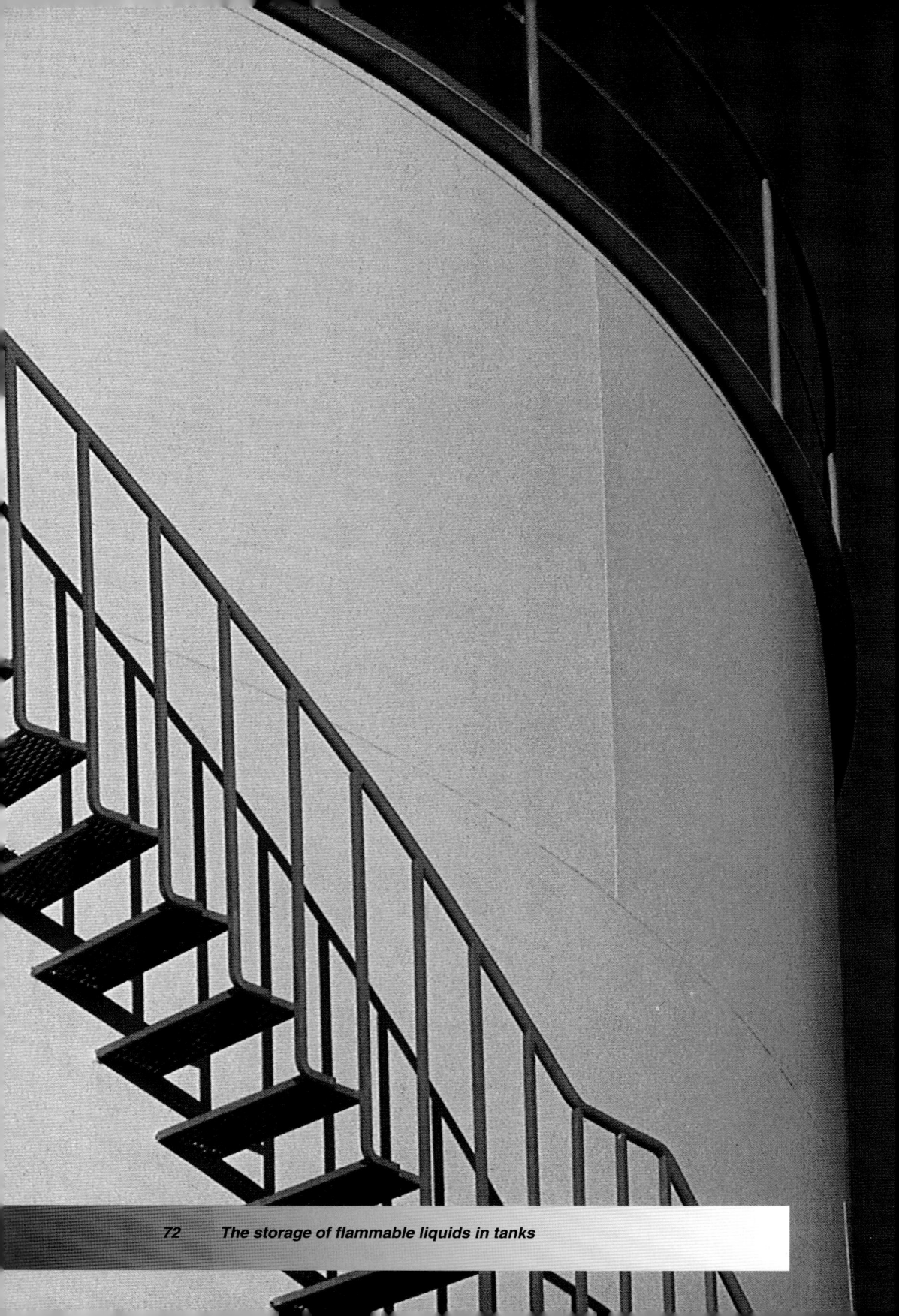

The storage of flammable liquids in tanks

REFERENCES

1   *Management of Health and Safety at Work Regulations 1992* SI 1992/2051
    HMSO 1992 ISBN 0 11 025051 6

2   *Management of health and safety at work. Management of Health and Safety at
    Work Regulations 1992. Approved Code of Practice* L21 HSE Books 1992
    ISBN 0 7176 0412 8

3   *5 steps to risk assessment* INDG163 HSE Books 1994 ISBN 0 7176 0904 9

4   *Health and Safety at Work etc Act 1974* Ch 37 HMSO 1974
    ISBN 0 10 543774 3

5   *A guide to the Health and Safety at Work etc Act 1974* L1 HSE Books 1992
    ISBN 0 7176 0441 1

6   *The Health and Safety (Enforcing Authority) Regulations 1989* SI 1989/1903
    HMSO 1989 ISBN 0 11 097903 6

7   *The Highly Flammable Liquids and Liquefied Petroleum Gases Regulations
    1972* SI 1972/917 HMSO 1972 ISBN 0 11 020917 6

8   *The storage of flammable liquids in containers* HSG51 HSE Books 1998
    ISBN 0 7176 1471 9

9   *The safe use and handling of flammable liquids* HSG140 HSE Books 1996
    ISBN 0 7176 0967 7

10 *Safe working with flammable substances* INDG227L HSE Books 1996
    ISBN 0 7176 1154 X

11 *Lift trucks in potentially flammable atmospheres* HSG113 HSE Books 1996
    ISBN 0 7176 0706 2

12 Institute of Petroleum *Marketing safety code: model code of safe practice
part 2* Heyden 1978 ISBN 0 8550 1322 2

13 Institute of Petroleum *Refining safety code: model code of safe practice part 3*
Heyden 1981 ISBN 0 85501 663 9

14 *Petroleum (Consolidation) Act 1928* Chapter 32 HMSO 1928

15 *Petroleum (Mixtures) Order 1929* HMSO 1929 ISBN 0 11 100031 9

16 *The Chemicals (Hazard Information and Packaging for Supply) Regulations 1994*
SI 1994/3247 HMSO 1994 ISBN 0 11 043877 9 as amended by *The Chemicals (Hazard
Information and Packaging for Supply) (Amendment) Regulations 1996* SI 1996/1092
HMSO 1996 ISBN 0 11 054570 2 and *The Chemicals (Hazard Information and
Packaging for Supply) (Amendment) Regulations 1997* SI 1997/1460 HMSO 1997
ISBN 0 11 063750 X

17 *Safety datasheets for substances and preparations dangerous for supply.
Guidance on regulation 6 of the Chemicals (Hazard Information and
Packaging for Supply) Regulations 1994. Approved Code of Practice* L62 HSE
Books 1994 ISBN 0 7176 0859 X

18 *Approved supply list. Information approved for the classification and labelling of
substances and preparations dangerous for supply. CHIP 96 and 97* L76
HSE Books 1997 ISBN 0 7176 1412 3

19 *Approved guide to the classification and labelling of substances and preparations
dangerous for supply. CHIP 97* L100 HSE Books 1997 ISBN 0 7176 0860 3

20 *CHIP 2 for everyone* HSG126 HSE Books 1995 ISBN 0 7176 0857 3

21 *Dispensing petrol: assessing and controlling the risk of fire and explosion at sites where
petrol is stored and dispensed as a fuel* HSG146 HSE Books 1996 ISBN 0 7176 1048 9

22 *The storage of LPG at fixed installations* HSG34 HSE Books 1987
ISBN 0 11 883908 X (currently under revision)

23 *The loading and unloading of bulk flammable liquids and gases at harbours and
inland waterways* GS40 HSE Books 1986 ISBN 0 11 883931 4 (currently under revision)

24 International Chamber of Shipping *International safety guide for oil tankers and
terminals (Isgott)* Witherby 1996 ISBN 1 85 6090817 8

25 *Environmental Protection Act 1990* HMSO 1990 ISBN 0 10 544390 5

26 *The Environmental Protection (Duty of Care) Regulations 1991* SI 1991/2839
    HMSO 1991 ISBN 0 11 015853 9

27 *Environmental Protection Act 1990 Part I Processes prescribed for air pollution control*
    by local enforcing authorities. Secretary of State's guidance - processes for the storage,
    loading and unloading of petrol at terminals PG1/13(96) HMSO ISBN 0 11 753348 3

28 *The Control of Substances Hazardous to Health Regulations 1994* SI 1994/3246
    HMSO 1994 ISBN 0 11 043721 7

29 *General COSHH ACOP (Control of Carcinogenic Substances) and Biological Agents*
    ACOP (Control of Biological Agents). Control of Substances Hazardous to Health
    Regulations 1994. Approved Codes of Practice L5 HSE Books 1995 ISBN 0 7176 0819 0

30 *Occupational exposure limits* EH 40/98 HSE Books 1998 ISBN 0 7176 1474 3

31 *The Control of Industrial Major Accident Hazards Regulations 1984* SI 1984/1902
    HMSO 1984 ISBN 0 11 047902 5

32 *A guide to the Control of Industrial Major Accident Hazards Regulations 1984*
    HSR21 HSE Books 1990 ISBN 011 885579 4

33 *The Control of Industrial Major Accident Hazards Regulations 1984 (CIMAH): Further*
    guidance on emergency plans HSG25 HSE Books 1985 ISBN 0 11 883831 8

34 *Electrical apparatus for explosive atmospheres Part 10 Classification of hazardous areas*
    BS EN 60079-10: 1996

35 Institute of Petroleum *Area classification code for petroleum installations: model code of*
    safe practice part 15 Wiley 1990 ISBN 0 47 192160 2

36 *Code of practice for the selection, installation and maintenance of electrical apparatus*
    for use in potentially explosive atmospheres (other than mining applications or explosive
    processing or manufacture) BS 5345 (in eight parts)

37 Institute of Petroleum *Fire precautions at petroleum refineries and bulk storage*
    installations: model code of safe practice part 19 Wiley 1993 ISBN 0 471 94328 2

38 *The keeping of LPG in cylinders and similar containers* CS4 HSE Books 1986
    ISBN 0 7176 0631 7 (currently under revision)

39 *Code of practice for ventilation principles and designing for natural ventilation*
    BS 5925: 1991

40 *Carbon steel welded horizontal cylindrical storage tanks* BS 2594: 1975

41 *Manufacture of vertical steel welded non-refrigerated storage tanks with butt-welded shells for the petroleum industry* BS 2654: 1989

42 *Design and construction of vessels and tanks in reinforced plastics* BS 4994: 1987

43 *Glass reinforced plastic vessels and tanks: advice to users* PM75 HSE Books 1991 ISBN 0 11 885608 1

44 *Road and rail tanker hose and hose assemblies for petroleum products, including aviation fuels* BS 3492: 1987

45 *Specification for the design and manufacture of site-built, vertical, cylindrical, flat-bottomed, above-ground, welded, metallic tanks for the storage of liquids at ambient temperature* prEN 265001 (draft not yet issued for public consultation - contact British Standards Institution for details)

46 *Underground tanks of glass-reinforced plastics (GRP) - Horizontal cylindrical tanks for the non-pressure storage of liquid petroleum based fuels* prEN 976
    Part 1: Requirements and test methods for single wall tanks
    Part 2: Transport, handling, storage and installation of single wall tanks
    Part 3: Requirements and test methods for double wall tanks
    Part 4: Transport, handling, storage and installation of double wall tanks

47 *Code of practice for protective coating of iron and steel structures against corrosion* BS 5493: 1977

48 *Cathodic protection Part 1 Code of practice for land and marine operations* BS 7361: Part 1 1991

49 *Bitumen-based coatings for cold application, suitable for use in contact with potable water* BS 3416: 1991

50 *Bitumen-based coatings for cold application, excluding use in contact with potable water* BS 6949: 1991

51 *Process piping* ASME B31.3-1996 American Society of Mechanical Engineers 1996

52 *Supplement 153 to ASME B31.3* Engineering Equipment and Materials Users Association (14/15 Belgrave Square, London SW1X 8PS Tel: 0171 235 5316/7) (updated annually)

53 *Pipe supports* BS 3974 (in three parts)

54 *Control of undesirable static electricity Part 2 Recommendations for particular industrial situations* BS 5958: Part 2 1991

55 *Testing of valves Part 2 Specification for fire type-testing requirements*
    BS 6755: Part 2 1987

56 Institute of Petroleum *Guidelines for the design and operation of gasoline
    vapour emission controls* Institute of Petroleum 1992 ISBN 0 85293 105 0

57 *Code of practice for protection of structures against lightning* BS 6651: 1992

58 *Venting atmospheric and low-pressure storage tanks (non-refrigerated and refrigerated)*
    API 2000 American Petroleum Institute 1992

59 *Fire tests on building materials and structures* BS 476 (in various parts)

60 *Code of practice for fire precautions in the chemical and allied industries* BS 5908: 1990

61 *Code of practice for earthing* BS 7430: 1991

62 *Health and Safety (Safety Signs and Signals) Regulations 1996* SI 1996/341
    HMSO 1996 ISBN 0 11 054093 X

63 *Lighting at work* HSG38 HSE Books 1997 ISBN 0 7176 1232 5

64 *Safety in pressure testing* GS4 HSE Books 1992 ISBN 0 7176 0811 5

65 *Oil burning equipment Part 5 Oil storage tanks* BS 799: Part 5 1987

66 *Code of practice for oil firing* BS 5410 (in three parts)

67 *Design and construction of ferrous piping installations for and in connection with land
    boilers* BS 806 (in various parts)

68   *Electrical surface heating* (in three parts) BS 6351

69 Institute of Petroleum *Code of practice for road tank vehicles equipped for bottom
    loading and vapour recovery* Institute of Petroleum 1987

70 *Carriage of Dangerous Goods by Road Regulations 1996* SI 1996/2095 HMSO 1996
    ISBN 0 11 062926 4

71 *Approved carriage list: information approved for the carriage of dangerous goods by
    road and rail other than explosives and radioactive material. Carriage of Dangerous
    Goods (Classification, Packaging and Labelling) and Use of Transportable Pressure
    Receptacles Regulations 1996. Carriage of Dangerous Goods by Road Regulations.
    Carriage of Dangerous Goods by Rail Regulations 1996* L90 HSE Books 1996
    ISBN 07176 1223 6

72 *Approved requirements and test methods for the classification and packaging of dangerous goods for carriage. Carriage of Dangerous Goods (Classification, Packaging and Labelling) and Use of Transportable Pressure Receptacles Regulations 1996* L88 HSE Books 1996 ISBN 0 7176 1221 X

73 *Carriage of Dangerous Goods (Classification, Packaging and Labelling) and Use of Transportable Pressure Receptacles Regulations 1996* SI 1996/2092 HMSO ISBN 0 11 062923 X

74 *Carriage of Dangerous Goods by Rail Regulations 1996* SI 1996/2089 HMSO ISBN 0 11 062919 1

75 *The carriage of dangerous goods explained. Part 2 guidance for road vehicle operators and others involved in the carriage of dangerous goods by road* HSG161 HSE Books 1996 ISBN 0 7176 1253 8

76 *The Provision and Use of Work Equipment Regulations 1992* SI 1992/2932 HMSO 1992 ISBN 0 11 025849 5

77 *Guidance on permit-to-work systems in the petroleum industry* HSE Books 1997 ISBN 0 7176 1281 3

78 *The cleaning and gas freeing of tanks containing flammable residues* CS15 HSE Books 1997 ISBN 0 7176 1365 8

79 Institute of Petroleum *Tank cleaning safety code: model code of safe practice part 16* Institute of Petroleum 1996 ISBN 0 471 97096 4

80 *Work in confined spaces* INDG258 HSE Books 1997 ISBN 0 7176 1442 5

81 *Safe work in confined spaces* L101 HSE Books 1997 ISBN 0 7176 1405 0

82 APEA/IP *Code of practice for the design, construction and operation of petrol filling stations* Association for Petroleum & Explosives Adminstration/Institute of Petroleum

83 *Code of practice for demolition* BS 6187: 1982

84 *Fire Service Act 1947* HMSO 1947 ISBN 0 10 850109 4

85 *Fire extinguishing installations and equipment on premises* BS 5306 (various parts)

86 *Fire Precautions Act 1971* HMSO 1971 ISBN 0 10 544071 X

87   *Fire Precautions Act 1971. Guide to fire precautions in existing places of work that require a fire certificate. Factories, offices, shops and railway premises* HMSO 1993 ISBN 0 11 341079 4

88   *Fire Certificates (Special Premises) Regulations 1976* SI 1976/2003 HMSO 1976 ISBN 0 11 062003 8

89   *Fire extinguishing installations and equipment on premises* BS 5306
Part 1: 1976 *Hydrant systems, hose reels and foam inlets*
Part 3: 1985 *Code of practice for the selection, installation and maintenance of portable fire extinguishers*

90   *Fixed firefighting systems - hose systems Part 1 Hose reels with semi-rigid hose* BS EN 671-1 1995

91   *Compendium of fire safety data: number 2: Industrial and process fire safety* Fire Protection Association 1986

92   *Fire and related properties of industrial chemicals* Fire Protection Association 1972

93   *Factories Act 1961* Chapter 34 HMSO 1961 ISBN 0 10 850027 6

94   *The Equipment and Protective Systems Intended for Use in Potentially Explosive Atmospheres Regulations 1996* SI 1996/192 HMSO 1996 ISBN 0 11 0539990

95   *Electricity at Work Regulations 1989* SI 1989/635 HMSO 1989 ISBN 0 11 096635 X

96   *Electricity and flammable substances: a short guide for small businesses* Institution of Chemical Engineers 1989 ISBN 0 85 295250 3

97   *Notification of Installations Handling Hazardous Substances Regulations 1982* SI 1982/1357 HMSO 1982 ISBN 0 11 027357 5

98   *Planning (Hazardous Substances) Regulations 1992* SI 1992/656 HMSO 1992 ISBN 0 11 023656 4

99   *Dangerous Substances (Notification and Marking of Sites) Regulations 1990* SI 1990/304 HMSO 1990 ISBN 0 11 003304 3

100 *Notification and marking of sites. Dangerous Substances (Notification and Marking of Sites) Regulations 1990* HSR29 HSE Books 1990 ISBN 0 11 885435 6

101 *The Reporting of Injuries, Diseases and Dangerous Occurrences (RIDDOR) Regulations 1995* SI 1995/3163 HMSO 1995 ISBN 0 11 053751 3

102 *Flame arresters* HSG158 HSE Books 1997 ISBN 0 17176 1191 4

103 *Flame arresters for general use* BS 7244: 1990

The future availability and accuracy of the references listed in this publication cannot be guaranteed.

For details of how to obtain HSE publications see inside back cover.

British and European Standards are available from:

389 Chiswick High Road
London
W4 9AL
Tel: 0181 996 7000
Fax: 0181 996 7001

GLOSSARY

Auto-ignition temperature: The minimum temperature at which a material will ignite spontaneously under specified test conditions. Also referred to as the minimum ignition temperature.

Bund: An area surrounded by a bund wall in which liquid spillage is contained.

Combustible: Capable of burning in air when ignited.

Element of construction: Any wall, floor, ceiling, roof, door or window (including the frame) etc which forms part of a building, room or other enclosure.

Enforcing authority: The authority with responsibility for enforcing the Health and Safety at Work etc Act 1974[2] and other relevant statutory provisions.

Fire-resisting: A fire-resisting element of construction is one which would have at least the stated period of fire resistance (relating to integrity, insulation and stability/load bearing capacity as appropriate) if tested, from either side, in accordance with British Standard 476[30], Part 8: 1972 or Parts 20 to 23:1987. In addition:

- where two or more elements of construction together provide separation, the junction between them should be bonded or fire-stopped to prevent or retard the passage of flames or hot gases, thus giving effective fire separation between the rooms or spaces on either side;

- elements of construction should be such that their fire-resisting properties are not impaired by everyday wear and tear. Additional protection, for example crash barriers, reinforcing plates or wearing strips, may be required where mechanical damage is foreseeable;

- the standard of fire-resistance relevant to the storage of flammable liquids is that which will allow adequate time, in the event of fire, for the alarm to be raised, for people to escape and for fire-fighting to be put in hand. The standard is not intended to afford protection from a complete burn-out of the storage installation.

Fire wall: A wall, screen or partition erected in the open air to help protect a tank containing flammable liquid from heat radiating from a nearby fire. A fire wall should have the following features:

- it should have no holes in it;

- it should have at least half-hour fire resistance;

- it should be weather-resistant; and

- it should be sufficiently robust to withstand foreseeable accidental damage.

A concrete, masonry or brick construction is recommended.

Flame arrester: A device to be fitted to the opening of an enclosure or to the connecting pipework of a system of enclosures and whose intended function is to allow flow but prevent flames from being transmitted. Most flame arresters consist of an assembly containing narrow passages or apertures through which gases or vapours can flow but which are too small for a flame to pass through[102,103].

Flammable: Capable of burning with a flame.

Flammable liquid: For the purpose of this book, flammable liquid means a liquid with a flashpoint of 55°C or below and stored at a near atmospheric pressure, except a liquid which has a flashpoint equal to or more than 21°C and less than or equal to 55°C and, when tested at 55°C in the manner described in Schedule 2 of the Highly Flammable Liquids and Liquefied Petroleum Gases Regulations 1972[3], does not support combustion.

Flammable range: The concentration of a flammable vapour in air falling between the upper and lower explosion limits.

Flashpoint: The minimum temperature at which a liquid, under specific test conditions, gives off sufficient flammable vapour to ignite momentarily on the application of an ignition source.

Hazard: Anything with the potential for causing harm. The harm may be to people, property or the environment, and may result from substances, machines, methods of work or work organisation.

Hazardous area: An area where flammable or explosive gas, or vapour-air mixtures (often referred to as explosive gas-air mixtures) are, or may be expected to be, present in quantities which require special precautions to be taken against the risk of ignition.

Hot work: This includes welding or the use of any equipment likely to cause flame, sparks or heat.

Impounding basin: An enclosure for collecting liquid spillage from one or more sources.

Incendive: Having sufficient energy to ignite a flammable mixture.

Inert: Incapable of supporting combustion; to render incapable of supporting combustion.

Interceptor: An installation to remove flammable liquid from aqueous effluents.

Lower explosion limit (LEL): The minimum concentration of vapour in air below which the propagation of a flame will not occur in the presence of an ignition source. Also referred to as the lower flammable limit or the lower explosive limit.

Non-combustible material: A material that fulfils the criteria for non-combustibility given in BS 476[30] Part 4: 1970. Alternatively, a material which, when tested in accordance with BS 476 Part 11: 1982, does not flame and gives no rise in temperature on either the centre or furnace thermocouples.

Permit-to-work: A document issued by an authorised person to permit work to be carried out safely in a defined area under specified conditions.

Risk: The likelihood that, should an incident occur, harm from a particular hazard will affect a specified population. Risk reflects both the likelihood that harm will occur and its severity in relation to the numbers of people who might be affected, and the consequences to them.

Risk assessment: The process of identifying the hazards present in any undertaking (whether arising from work activities or other factors) and those likely to be affected by them, and of evaluating the extent of the risks involved, bearing in mind whatever precautions are already being taken.

Underground tank: A tank buried in the ground so that no part of the tank is above ground except for fittings attached to the tank.

Upper explosion limit (UEL): The maximum concentration of vapour in air above which the propagation of a flame will not occur. Also referred to as the upper flammable limit or the upper explosive limit.

Vapour: The gaseous phase released by evaporation from a material that is a liquid at normal temperatures and pressure.

Zone: The classified part of a hazardous area, representing the probability of a flammable vapour (or gas) and air mixture being present.

Printed in the UK for the Health and Safety Executive   1/98   C80